Research Degrees for
Health Professionals

Research Degrees for Health Professionals

Richard Hays MBBS PhD MD FRACGP FACRRM

Professor of Medical Education
School of Medicine
Keele University
United Kingdom

Radcliffe Publishing
Oxford • New York

Radcliffe Publishing Ltd
18 Marcham Road
Abingdon
Oxon OX14 1AA
United Kingdom

www.radcliffe-oxford.com
Electronic catalogue and worldwide online ordering facility.

British Library Cataloguing in Publication Data

A catalogue record for this book is available from the British Library.

ISBN-13: 978 1 84619 127 5

Typeset by Phoenix Photosetting, Chatham, Kent
Printed and bound by TJI Digital, Padstow, Cornwall

Contents

Preface

A great part, I believe, of the Art is to be able to observe.

Hippocrates 460–357 BC

This book is for all those poor souls who feel an inclination to undertake further education and is written in a way that answers questions relevant to their work. By definition, this target audience is those with at least an undergraduate coursework degree and with at least some work experience in their chosen profession. While any postgraduate education can enhance career development, the kind of education with the most potential to lead practitioners to the leading edge of their professions is research training.

Research training does not need to be seen as daunting. There is a wide range of research training available, from lower level coursework modules through to higher level, research project-based programmes, many of them designed for full-time study. Few practising health professionals have the time or the inclination to suspend professional work and study full-time, and so embark on complex pathways that combine research and professional practice. The choice of pathways is potentially confusing and there are numerous challenges to reaching a satisfactory outcome and maintaining sanity.

Unlike research student handbooks, most of which are written for full-time students straight out of Bachelor level degrees, this book adopts the perspective of busy professionals who balance part-time research within busy lives. It therefore assumes that research is not the only focus and describes how to survive, perhaps even thrive, in a complex situation. The information provided is no less relevant to full-time research students, particularly more mature students, who also balance work and personal pressures.

With careful planning, prediction of potential pressure points, and early detection of challenges and intervention, research training even amidst complex lives, can be very rewarding and even life-changing.

Richard Hays
July 2007

7

About the author

Richard Hays began his medical career as a rural general practitioner in Australia. After 10 years of full-time practice, he almost accidentally entered academic life, spurred on by questions arising from his part-time teaching post to which he could not easily find answers. Much to his surprise he gained a research degree in education while running a general practice. He then continued to ask and answer questions as he followed opportunities in teaching and education research at both postgraduate and undergraduate levels.

From 1999 to 2005 he guided the development of a new Australian School of Medicine (James Cook University), where there is a focus on regional and rural healthcare issues. He is now Head of the School of Medicine at Keele University, with responsibility for guiding the development of a new curriculum. He has a strong record of achievement in research and publishing, authoring about 100 research papers, and several books, covering his major interests in faculty development, assessment methodology and quality of clinical and education service delivery. One of his most enjoyable tasks is supervising others choosing to conduct research in applied healthcare settings.

Case studies

Throughout this book references will be made to progress on three evolving case studies that demonstrate how health professionals with a varied range of experience and interests approach research that is relevant to their professional roles.

Case A

Jamie is a GP who completed postgraduate vocational training about five years ago and is now established in a group practice that hosts both medical students and GP registrars. When the partner with primary responsibility for teaching wants to cut down hours, Jamie is asked to take over. He has always had some interest in teaching and says yes. He attends 'train the trainer' sessions and enrols in a 'teacher training' module at the local medical school, although this is about an hour away by road and attendance is difficult. Jamie is soon managing both one-to-one teaching in the practice and a group of six medical students in his 'teaching hub' practice. This is enjoyable, but Jamie is puzzled because sometimes sessions work out really well, while others do not seem to work well at all. Feedback from the students is collected regularly, but while generally positive, this is rather non-specific. Jamie begins to wonder: 'Why are these sessions so variable in their quality? What can I do to improve things?'

Case B

Ahmed is a registered nurse who recently completed a postgraduate certificate in emergency care nursing and now works only in a busy emergency department. After a few months working there, Ahmed notices that managing patient flows is often a major challenge to efficiency and quality of care provided. Particularly over weekends, when the department accepts a lot of medium-level urgency sporting injuries, mostly orthopaedic, but this impairs the capacity to manage the injuries from frequent road accidents on the nearby motorway. Ahmed begins to ask: 'Can we develop a better system for managing these sporting injuries in a timely way without affecting the capacity for managing serious trauma?'

Case C

Susan is a speech language therapist with 15 years experience in general professional practice, who has deepening interest and expertise in language and learning disorders in children and teenagers. Susan has completed a coursework masters level qualification in special education needs in childhood, and this provided extensive knowledge of a broad range of approaches and assessment tools. As a result, Susan is referred an increasing number of clients who pose challenges, such as adolescents with less well defined language and learning problems (e.g. dyslexia) and rather vague academic performance problems. Susan finds that most available assessment tools are not appropriate for these clients, as the tools were developed and standardised for younger, less academically able and less culturally diverse populations. Susan begins to ask: 'How can I provide a better, more culturally sensitive, evidence-based and more accurate service?'

Chapter 1

The relevance of research training

All the world is a laboratory to the inquiring mind.

Martin H Fischer 1944

Why even consider research training?

Professional careers usually commence with an undergraduate coursework degree. The increasing trend towards graduate entry professional degree programmes means that many will have more than one undergraduate coursework degree. These degrees are usually targeted at producing graduates who are fit to commence professional practice, often under some form of supervision, which may be formal and structured, leading to professional recognition and/or registration. As a rule, undergraduate degrees are designed to produce graduates with certain core competencies that span both academic and professional aspects. That is, there are generic academic skills that bachelor level degrees are required to provide, and there are certain core competencies that professions require. The former are more concerned with thinking and basic knowledge, and the latter with application of knowledge and professional skills as a novice professional. Neither sets of learning outcomes imply a post-basic level of mastery.

Being a professional means a lifetime of continuing professional development. Requirements for postgraduate education vary between professions, but at a minimum all professionals are required to maintain currency of practice. Currency of practice is a rather complex concept that combines maintenance of previously acquired knowledge and skills, acquisition of necessary new knowledge and skills, and the judgement about how and when to apply both new and old in a way that achieves high quality practice.

At this level, academic and professional education diverges, offering opportunities and pathways that have strong differences, and yet often overlap. Traditional continuing professional development either adds depth, as in narrowing the scope to a specialty, or provides continuous updates for current scope of practice. Some include research components, but the main focus is on application of knowledge and skills within the professional context.

Postgraduate academic training really means further development of thinking skills and builds towards research training. Masters level programmes used to always include some research component, and doctoral level degrees always meant a substantially or entirely research-based experience. This traditional approach has changed, such that some higher level degrees no longer involve research, and some university degrees include more professional, rather than just academic, content. There are now many variations on what is offered, each designed to meet a particular need or market (see Chapter 2). Most postgraduate degrees are provided on a user pays basis, some with high fees.

So, back to the question. Given that all professionals must maintain currency of practice, and therefore must participate in continuing professional development, why would anyone consider research training?

What can research training add, and what can it not add?

Possible answers to these questions are listed in Box 1.1; each of these is a potential outcome of embarking on a research pathway. Promotion may well be an outcome of continuing professional development of any kind, but research training is perhaps the least likely pathway for professionals to achieve promotion quickly, as research training is at least initially a different career direction. Similarly, income is unlikely to rise in a hurry, and may well fall, as professional activities are often better remunerated than academic pursuits. Fame is possible, but probably only following a long and distinguished career, unless the research training leads to truly ground-breaking research outcomes.

Box 1.1 Reasons for considering postgraduate education.

- Improve promotion prospects
- Increase personal satisfaction
- Increase income
- Increase recognition
- Facilitate career change
- Complement current career

Most tangible rewards are longer term, and unpredictable. Research training may be more relevant to career change, as a combination of professional and academic training can produce a different kind of person, who may develop a broader set of skills to those who remain in narrower professional life. People who successfully combine the two may be highly sought after for key leadership roles within their profession, as they may demonstrate high level understanding of how to apply theory into professional practice. This is not a guaranteed, or even necessarily a desirable, outcome for many. These issues are discussed in more detail in the final chapter.

The most important reason to consider undertaking research training is personal satisfaction. People who find themselves asking questions about 'why' and 'how' things are as they appear may well enjoy working out the answers. Research training can improve the capacity to find answers to such questions. Those of us who do this generally derive deep satisfaction from the problem solving process. The level of interest and satisfaction is probably related to personality. Readers of this book may already know deep down that they are interested in answering at least 'a' question of relevance to their professional life.

Those who want to better understand their own personality may learn something from exercises such as a learning styles questionnaire, which can help individuals understand how they prefer to learn (there are several)[1, 2] or the Myers Briggs Type Indicator (MBTI), which can identify the preferred ways that individuals think and process information.[3] While there is not any 'better' learning style or personality profile, and anybody can adapt and succeed in whatever they choose to do, it is interesting that academics tend to have particular learning styles (enjoying theory, reflection and understanding) and are over-represented in certain MBTI profiles (intuitive thinkers who draw strength from reflection).

Pathways to research training

Broadly speaking, there are two pathways to research training. The most common is where graduates from bachelor degrees proceed rapidly to masters and doctoral level programmes with little or no 'outside' (of university) work experience. This is the model that universities and academics understand and support best. Bright minds are identified young and nurtured by academic role models who place students in their research teams and mentor their progress. Early research funding is almost guaranteed from the host team, as projects usually form part of the broader research programme of the supervisors. Publications are also almost guaranteed, as research students are included in report writing teams, although usually not as the primary authors. Grant writing skills will be learned as the team will be in a more or less constant state of grant submission to sustain their research programme.

These 'early' research students tend to have simpler personal life arrangements. As they are younger, they are less likely to have dependent partners and children, or expensive mortgages. They may be more mobile, able to move towns and universities to pursue research interests and supervisors. They will not have had the chance to become accustomed to higher salaries. In many ways this pathway is a continuation of the undergraduate life, relatively low earning but very stimulating and enjoyable.

By their mid-twenties, these students may well have a PhD, successful research grant applications, and several published papers. They are however, unlikely to have professional training and life experience outside universities. They rarely have any job security for several years, as they live from grant to grant, and then post-doctoral fellowships – all so-called 'soft' money – as success depends on high performance within a very competitive research world. Depending on the level of success through this period, they may establish themselves as 'independent' researchers, with a team of their own, and go on to have very successful research careers. Because of the narrow and intense focus on research built on basic sciences, the research is usually not particularly relevant to applied professional research, although occasionally these early researchers join more applied professional research teams from the beginning of their research training.

The other model is more common in the health professions, and is less understood by universities. Most health professional students choose their course with more of a focus on their chosen vocation, and are keen to get to the point of almost guaranteed employment and income generation. Further pressure comes from the longer duration of professional courses, compared to other undergraduate degrees, resulting in higher student debt at graduation. Finally, the potential for research related directly to their chosen vocation is lower until graduates have an opportunity to gain experience in the professional workplace. Hence interest in research often comes later to health professionals.

Common characteristics of this group of research students are listed in Box 1.2.

Box 1.2 Characteristics of health professional research students.

- Usually more mature
- Usually more complex personal lives
- Usually greater financial problems
- Interests usually more applied than basic
- More likely to be seeking interesting career enhancement

The first group of characteristics relate to the greater maturity of these students. They are more likely to have partners and dependent children, bigger debts, and other family complications such as ill parents. If they have a mortgage, they will also be less free to move for study, and so will explore local options. They will find the fall in income that is almost inevitable when replacing professional income generating time with research time, that may earn little or no income, very difficult. However, maturity means not just older (on average), but also having a different approach to learning. They are more likely to behave in the manner described as *adult learners*, meaning that they will want to be more in control of their learning,[4] by choosing a research pathway that is more relevant to their professional lives.

The second group of characteristics is that their research interests are usually more *applied* than *basic* in nature. Applied research is that which builds on basic sciences to research about more contextually and professionally relevant issues. For example, while basic research might consider the possible neurotransmitter imbalance in depression, applied research will look at the effectiveness of neuro-transmitter therapy plus psychotherapy. Their potential research questions are more likely to have come from professional practice, and even from personal encounters and experiences. There may be a greater desire to produce evidence that explains and/or informs professional practice. Depending on the stage of their career, they are also more likely to be considering some form of change in career direction, more likely building on and enhancing a somewhat diver-sified career in the current profession, but in some cases a more dramatic change, perhaps including being an academic in their professional discipline.

These differences have several implications for those wishing to undertake, and those agreeing to supervise, more applied professional research degrees. The process can be simpler, more complex, or a combination of both, depending on the partic-ular circumstances. What is certain is that the process is different from that of the usual research supervision model. Both students and supervisors need to be aware of these differences, and their implications, which are listed in Table 1.1.

These implications are the basis of the following chapters, which guide readers through the process of undertaking a research project based on a question that emerges from professional practice. Issues are explored using three examples of potential research questions that recur in each chapter as specific issues are dealt

Table 1.1 Implications for health professional research degrees.

Student profile	Supervisor skills
Part-time, maintaining professional practice	Accommodate greater flexibility
Wanting control over research topic and process	Provide 'softer touch' guidance
Having large, diffuse research questions	Guide refinement of answerable questions
Having a weak methodology knowledge	Focus on guiding learning of methodology
Coming with no formal project funding	Help identify potential research funding
Underestimating the importance of disseminating results	Promote and support dissemination

with. This approach allows readers to work through the issues with both concrete examples and opportunities to consider in parallel their own research ideas. This more 'case based' approach is common in health professional education, and is equally relevant to postgraduate research training.

Case studies

Jamie, Ahmed and Susan are at the stage where they have identified reasonably broad professional development needs. In theory, all such needs could be addressed through attending some kind of training course, and our three colleagues make enquiries about what is available.

Case A: Variable quality of learning strategies

Jamie asks the people running the teacher training course and is told that they do not have a module that specifically looks at his question. They also do not know of any other courses that are likely to deal with such a broad question. 'That may be a research question!' is the smiling reply. They advise enrolling in their Certificate of Medical Education course, as this may provide further knowledge and skills that might help him build his experience. Jamie agrees, as such a path fits relatively easily with his complex work requirements, but deep down wonders if he should not find a way of satisfying his need to focus on (to him) the specific question in his mind. He knows that the Certificate course does not include research methods, but he did a small research project as an undergraduate student and feels that he will be able to refresh and revise that knowledge when he needs to, as he is interested in only a small and simple project.

Case B: Effective triaging of sporting injuries

Ahmed asks his supervisor for advice, and is told that while the idea is interesting, they are all much too busy to be able to do anything about it. He looks outside the hospital for courses that might help, but a search of websites of professional organisations and universities reveals nothing that appears to be related. He next approaches one of the nurse tutors from the local university, and is referred to one of the senior lecturers on the main campus. This person is very helpful, and suggests that Ahmed enrol in the postgraduate academic programme, such as their diploma/masters course, as this might provide some ideas about how to answer the question, even if it does not directly answer it. Ahmed has had very limited exposure to research so far in his training, and is pleased that the diploma/masters course includes some research methodology components.

Case C: A better, more culturally sensitive, evidence-based and more accurate service

Susan is, in academic terms, perhaps the most advanced of the three. She has already completed a masters level course, and that included modules on research methods, although not necessarily the methods she might have to use for her project. She recognises that her question could be framed as a research question concerning standardising either current or newly developed assessment tools for her target populations, and that might need some additional research methodology expertise. Susan does a literature review on the topic and is not surprised to discover that there is very little there. She contacts the masters course director at her university and asks about the possibility of conducting some kind of part-time research project.

Each of our three colleagues has to make a decision on where to go next. It is quite possible for such questions to arise from time to time, depending on current interests, and for interest to wane under the burden of professional and personal demands; not every interesting idea from professional practice can be followed up! Some might decide to follow that more individual, less formal approach to research, and not worry too much about achieving a high quality outcome; curiosity can be satisfied with less than that. On the other hand, the decision may be to follow a more formal path that provides academic support, a higher chance of a high quality outcome, and some form of qualification. If the latter is decided, then the next step for Jamie, Ahmed and Susan is to seek advice from an experienced researcher in an academic institution about how to address the broad research questions each has identified.

Conclusion

Health professionals with research interests usually follow a career path that is different from those in other academic disciplines and therefore often acquire research training in different ways. Most commence research training with professional clinical experience, choose to research topics of personal interest that are related to their professional practice, and undertake the research part-time. This requires a different approach to that of younger, full-time research students and their supervisors. Following chapters explore through the three case studies a model of research supervision that is more appropriate for health professional research training, with the aim of making research training more accessible to health professionals who wish to continue to provide professional clinical services.

References

1   Mumford A, Honey P. Questions and answers on the Learning Styles Questionnaire. Industrial and Commercial Training: 1992; 24 (see http://www.emeraldinsight.com/Insight/ac_FullTextOptions.do?contentId=837961&contentType=Article).

2   Bligh J. The S-SDLRS: a short questionnaire about self-directed learning. *Postgrad Educ General Pract.* 1993; **4**: 121–5.

3   Myers-Briggs Type Indicator: see www.myersbriggs.org

4   Knowles M. *The Adult Learner: A Neglected Species.* 3rd ed. Houston Tx: Gulf Publishing Company; 1984.

Chapter 2

Choosing from the variety of research training programmes

So-called original research is now regarded as a profession, adopted by hundreds of men, and communicated by a system of training.

William Stanley Jevons 1835–82

The spectrum of postgraduate research training opportunities

One of the certainties of postgraduate education, including postgraduate research training, is that there are many ways of reaching goals. In deciding which pathway to choose, the most important question to ask, and answer, is: Why am I doing this?

There are several possible answers to this question. If the answer is to dabble and follow a rather unhurried, personal research journey, without achieving any formal recognition, then it may be possible to simply follow a self-directed journey of identifying questions, choosing a method, doing the research (often self-funded) and then deciding what to do with the results. This is a style that suits many independent professional people as it fits best into complex lives, but it has major potential disadvantages. Novice researchers commonly have difficulty refining an answerable research issue or question that has already been addressed. They are unlikely to have any real background in research methodology, and so may either not apply the most appropriate methods to the issue or question, or apply appropriate methods poorly. They may also not be concerned about reporting interesting and relevant results in appropriate academic and/or professional outlets. A common result is that, while individuals can have an enjoyable time on this pathway, they may well waste time and personal funds by not producing a credible, reported outcome.

Should the answer be to receive at least some formal research advice and support, then there are two choices. The first is to combine the self-directed path described above with some informal contact with one or more professional researchers. This can add the academic rigour to provide a credible outcome, without the pressure of institutional time-frames and requirements, but has two disadvantages. The first is that it may be hard to find academics who can provide the necessary degree of support, as this is an informal arrangement that fits poorly into busy academic life, where there is generally little 'spare' time. The only potential reward for academics providing informal assistance is a name on resulting publications, and that requires a high quality research project. This is of course possible, but is less likely. The second disadvantage is that there will be little or no formal reward for what might be very useful and satisfying work.

The second choice is to seek formal research advice and training from experienced academic researchers. This again carries several choices, linked to the level of the degree programme; the usual broad academic categories are listed in Table 2.1. The choice may depend on the level of commitment to research training, the time available, the balance of potentially competing pressures, and access issues, such as geographic location of courses. If in doubt, it may be better to commence with modest ambitions, to gain a more informed idea of what might be involved. A sample experience is a reasonable basis for further planning and involvement, and it is possible to 'upgrade' time commitment and the scale of training.

Some brief explanation is necessary of the range of courses included in Table 2.1. There are two kinds of degree programmes, although the two models often overlap. The first is coursework-based degree programmes. Most of these include little or no research training up to diploma level, although most at masters and doctoral levels do include at least some research training. A more recent development is the professional doctorate, which is usually like a masters level programme, only longer and to a deeper level. Most masters and doctoral level coursework degrees include some component of research training, but less so than research-based masters and PhD degrees. However, some more recent

Table 2.1 The range of postgraduate training courses.

Coursework-based	Research project-based
Postgraduate certificate	Masters degree
Postgraduate diploma	Doctorate
Masters degree	
Doctorate	

Table 2.2 Postgraduate research programmes.

	Duration (Full-time equivalence)	Supervised	Research component
Coursework masters	2 years	Yes	Nil to minor, probably limited to proposal, literature review
Research masters	2 years	Yes	Moderate to substantial, not necessarily a new topic
Professional doctorate	2–3 years	Yes	Nil to substantial, part of a portfolio of diverse tasks
Doctor of Philosophy	2–4 years	Yes	Substantial, a new research topic
Higher doctorate	N/A	No	A body of published research indicating a major contribution

masters and doctoral level programmes do not include any research training, so if research training is the goal, read the programme information carefully. Those wanting to move into formal academic career tracks need to be very careful here, as non-research based masters and doctorate level degrees may not carry the same academic respect as research-based doctorates. If in doubt, seek advice from academic colleagues.

The second kind of degree programme is the traditional, research project-based programme that at completion can lead to a change to a more academic career, as they are regarded as the baseline academic qualifications for academic health professionals. A summary of both coursework and research-based programmes is provided in Table 2.2.

Coursework-based degree programmes

Many health professionals will have completed some form of research task during their undergraduate course, and so most have some research training, but this is far below that required of doctoral level research. Hence proceeding directly to a doctoral research programme is not wise, unless further research achievement has been gained through postgraduate research experience. Some achieve this informally through applying good ideas with sound advice from more experienced researchers, but for many the easiest entry point is via a postgraduate coursework programme. Most of these are 'tiered' programmes, such that an individual can exit with a postgraduate certificate, postgraduate diploma, masters or doctoral level degree, depending on the duration of study and the number of subjects studied. Entering students usually commence with subjects that allow exploration of professional practice through a range of conceptual frameworks, a process that provides a foundation for achieving better understanding of their professional practice. This can be both personally and professionally satisfying, and may be useful for thinking about becoming a teacher of either undergraduate or postgraduate students within the profession. At completion of either the certificate or diploma level, individuals may continue with predominantly professional practice, or can progress to masters degree level training.

At masters level, the focus usually narrows and the intensity increases, although more optional subjects should be available to cater for a wide range of interests. Formal research methods modules are usually included, and some programmes will also include either small- or moderate-sized research tasks, or even a modest-scale research project. Those who complete a coursework masters degree should have demonstrated mastery of some quantitative and/or qualitative research methods, and will be capable of making a significant contribution to academic professional practice, even if they do not subsequently complete a doctoral level programme. At completion of a coursework masters programme, graduates with some research training should be eligible to enrol in a PhD programme.

Coursework doctorates are a relatively recent and controversial initiative that is said to have first appeared in the USA. The academic title 'doctor' has traditionally meant achievement in research training, and academic institutions are wary of degrees that reward broader, rather than 'higher', academic achievement with that title. However, they are becoming more popular and more widely available. In concept they are simply a longer, broader and perhaps deeper version of a coursework masters degree, and generally offer subjects that build on professional practice, although may include research methodology subjects. They may represent genuinely high achievement, but the quality is still regarded as being variable across institutions. The best advice is to enrol in a coursework professional doctorate at a reputable university.

Research project-based degree programmes

Research project-based programmes provide a more self-directed learning experience to a deeper level, where students build research training around a substantial research project that is supervised by one or more experienced researchers. Research degrees require more commitment by students, as much more is left to them to do personally. The degrees come in a variety of programmes, each with different expectations, workloads and outcomes, as summarised in Table 2.2. The lowest level of research project-based degree is the masters level. A research masters degree involves research that is not necessarily new, but might apply reported approaches in different contexts, and should result in a publication in a peer-reviewed journal. Where the masters programme is entirely research-based (i.e. no coursework, with a more substantial research project), it is often regarded as an honours masters degree. This higher masters level degree is now less popular, as while the standards and status are lower than for a PhD, the workload is sometimes not much less. It is therefore wise for an individual eligible for an entirely research-based degree programme (usually with a prior coursework masters degree) to seek advice about enrolling directly in PhD programmes, where for a modest increase in workload, time-frame and standards, the rewards are higher.

A doctoral level degree usually requires a larger research project, and a higher standard outcome/product. Doctorate level research degrees are often narrower than masters level research degrees, because students learn in greater depth about research methods relevant to only a particular research category. The exception to this is the research-based professional doctorate, which is broader, but is expected to achieve similar standards. PhD theses should achieve something genuinely new, requiring more familiarity with the literature, greater attention to research methods, greater care in reporting, longer theses, and (ideally) several peer-reviewed papers.

Research-based professional doctorates are unusual in that they reflect more than one research-based task, the results of which are submitted in a portfolio, rather than a single thesis. The tasks include a substantial research-based thesis component, perhaps comprising about half of the academic workload, but also can include minor research products. These might include published papers or conference presentations from other research projects, a monograph prepared for professional practice, book chapters or even a whole book. Monographs could include policy documents written for the workplace. All inclusions in the portfolio should reflect an ability to access, synthesise and build on research findings, as well as communicate academic material clearly via oral and written presentations. This can clearly be of the same standard as the 'usual' PhD outcomes, and offers the advantage of making the achievement more directly relevant to professional practice. As with coursework doctorates, choose the university carefully (see below).

All research degrees require supervision from one or more experienced researchers. Some supervisors may have successful research programmes that offer ready-made topics and resources, but it is more common for health professional research students to have their own research question to answer. At completion of a research masters or PhD programme, one is regarded as research trained, albeit in a narrow field.

Another kind of research degree offered by most universities is a higher doctorate. This is the highest form of academic recognition that can be bestowed for academic achievement. Merit is a judgement by external research peers, based on consideration of a submission of a substantial collection of published research over a period of time that is judged to contribute substantially to knowledge in the particular academic field. The submitted thesis does not require supervision of a research project and indeed ideally applicants already have a PhD. The degrees are called either Doctorates of Science (DSc) or Doctorates of Medicine (MD), depending on previous qualifications and the particular profession. Standards are high. Some universities enrol only their own bachelor level graduates or staff members to these courses. For novice researchers, this level is a long way off, but it may be useful to understand the complete hierarchy of research degrees.

Within the medical profession there is confusion over the MD degree, which currently exists in three forms. The first and most traditional is where recent medical graduates undertake specialist training and also conduct research, usually related to their specialty, submitting a thesis based on this research. This is usually unsupervised or only partly supervised, as it is assumed that medical students learned enough about research methods during their longer Bachelor degrees. However, while some of these MDs are of a very high standard, there is wide variation in quality and a high failure rate, partly because most medical students do not actually learn much about medical research during their first degree! Hence in some countries (for example Australia) this model has been discouraged, to be replaced by supervised PhD training. Universities in the UK are also replacing the traditional MD with either masters or professional doctorate programmes. Many of the MD programmes left operate under the same rules as PhD programmes, requiring supervision and greater uniformity; this is the second MD model. The third model is the higher doctorate, described above. This diversity makes the task of cv readers more complex, as the degree MD may mean anything from quite low to very high standards.

Choice of university

There are a lot of universities to choose from, many ways of considering their relative merits, and many ways of ranking them. While almost everybody has heard of Oxford, Cambridge, Harvard, Stanford, and the Sorbonne, only a tiny minority of university students attend such powerful and venerable institutions. No university is excellent at everything it offers, and so no single university is necessarily best in any national system for its courses.

The key issues in research training are: first, learn the basics of research methods; and second, for research projects choose the best supervisors you can connect with. For basic research training the choice of university is probably relatively unimportant, as any research-based university (not all of them are!)

will have a range of courses. The second issue – choice of supervisor for a research project – is more important, particularly for doctoral level projects, as good research supervisors with relevant content expertise are harder to find and can sometimes be in unexpected places. They will be in research-based universities, but often not the better known universities. A literature search will often identify the individual researchers publishing in relevant research areas, and from that look at the web pages of the universities that employ them.

In practice, many potential research students will choose a university with which they have some links. This may be from earlier studies or professional contacts in other settings. This approach is usually sound as a place to start, because good supervisors will recognise when assistance may be necessary from academics in other universities (see Chapter 5 on supervision). The higher the level of training (i.e. doctoral level), the greater the likely need for more expert advice.

Location of courses

Universities have a main base in a particular geographic location, but increasingly offer courses in flexible delivery mode, so that students do not necessarily have to be physically close. Many universities regard themselves as truly international institutions and brand names, and for some courses enrolling in one half a world away may work well. However, the degree to which support can be provided varies considerably, so it is advisable to carefully read institutional web pages and to seek advice from others enrolled in courses delivered from distant institutions. Most flexible delivery courses are coursework degrees, although at masters level these will usually include some research component. With entirely research degrees, the key issue to consider is ease of access to the supervisors, with whom there will have to be frequent discussions about methods and progress. This does not preclude a distant relationship, particularly if students are more experienced in research, students and supervisors know each other well, all parties are prepared to commit to frequent email/telephone contact, and some structured visits can be scheduled for deeper discussions over key issues.

Inexperienced researchers are more likely to need closer support, and should try harder to negotiate arrangements with relatively close universities. This decision may limit the scope of available supervision and support, but is probably a safer place to start. More experienced research students may be more concerned with finding the most appropriate supervisor expertise and may manage with a more distant relationship. Doctoral level research may benefit from supervision by an acknowledged international expert, and modern communications technology can allow this to work well. This issue is discussed further in Chapter 5.

Where to start

It may sound obvious, but novice researchers are most unlikely to be able to commence research training at doctoral level, and may struggle to start at the masters level without evidence of prior relevant coursework, such as research training modules. Although most health professional courses include components of research training and experience, these are usually both limited and highly supported, and so not sufficient to allow commencement of a higher level, more independent research project. However, whereas most entrants to postgraduate academic training would require an honours bachelor level degree, greater flexibility is usually allowed for health professionals where their bachelor level degree included research components.

Hence most health professionals with some practice experience and some early research training may be allowed to commence at the masters level. Depending on the level of their prior research training, they may be required to complete coursework subjects that provide basic research method training in quantitative methods, qualitative methods, or both.

The early discussions

All prospective research students, having decided to explore at least the possibility of undertaking research training to answer their research questions, need to obtain advice from an experienced researcher. The discussions with the experienced researcher will include consideration of the issues listed in Box 2.1.

Box 2.1 Questions to ask at early meetings.

1 What is the prior research training and experience of the potential research student?
2 Is there a clear question or issue?
3 What is the potential scale of the research that would be required to address the research question?
4 What is the level of commitment that the individual can make to the research?
5 What resources might be available to facilitate the research project?

The first question is about determining the capacity of the potential research student for commencing the relatively independent and self-driven process of a professional research degree. The higher the level of the proposed research training and degree, the greater the requirement for prior research training and experience, and the deeper that experience should be.

The second question is about defining whether or not there is even a research issue to address. A literature search is needed to work that out, as it will determine whether or not the issue has already been thought of or even answered. If there is some literature but the research has not been replicated enough times or in enough contexts to achieve a generalised answer, then the prospects for research increase. Should there be a genuine gap in the literature around the issue, then the prospects for higher level research increase.

The third question is about determining whether the potential research should be: an exploration of an interesting idea that might lead to a bigger project later (a 'pilot' project); a replication or adaptation of a documented research project in a different context; or a genuinely new issue that might lead to a unique contribution to the literature? The latter is required for doctoral level research.

The fourth and fifth questions are about ensuring that the research can succeed. The bigger and more complex the research project, the greater the need for substantial quarantined time over a considerable period, and for funding to make it happen. There also needs to be research supervisors with the appropriate and relevant research expertise. Research is most likely to be successful when it is planned carefully, and this is a crucial stage of the planning process. Research students and supervisors should proceed with projects only after consideration of these issues and agreement on how to proceed.

Case studies

Each of the case studies has an individual at a different level of experience. Jamie is the most likely to have done at least some formal research training during the basic medical degree, has professional clinical qualifications, and is training for a postgraduate certificate, which usually includes no research training. Ahmed has a postgraduate professional certificate, but probably little research training or experience. Susan has more years of professional experience and a coursework masters level qualification, and has a clearer research question.

Case A

Jamie finds the certificate in medical education interesting, in that it provides frameworks and evidence to support his experience and growing role as an educator. He enjoys the education role so much that he negotiates (with difficulty) a reduction in his clinical sessions and an increase in his education sessions. However, he is still not sure that he is much closer to answering his question. In fact, he has experiences with learners that make the question even more pressing. He would prefer to extend his training in the local university, with whose medical school he already has a relationship and where he has completed his certificate of medical education. He makes an appointment with the course director to see what else he could do.

Case B

Ahmed enrols in a postgraduate diploma course that is available in highly accessible web-based modules from a nursing school 100 miles away that has a reputation for strong distance education support. However he soon finds that neither of the modules he has studied have much to do with his question. He emails the senior lecturer to ask if there is a better way of doing this. The senior lecturer recognises that Ahmed's question is potentially a research question concerning clinical algorithms and management pathways, but says that it is not her area of expertise. Ahmed asks if the senior lecturer could ask around to see if there is someone who might know more about these issues.

Case C

For Susan the obvious choice of university is the same one where she studied for her coursework masters degree, as she knows the academic staff there and feels comfortable approaching them. Susan has a very constructive meeting with the course director, who agrees that pursuing a research path is appropriate. The meeting soon becomes a discussion of how to proceed.

Conclusion

Research ideas need to crystallise into achievable research projects. The level of the research degree training that is commenced depends on the prior research training and experience of the potential research student, the clarity of the question, the scale of the research project and the availability of required resources. It is unlikely that many potential research students will be able to commence at doctoral level, at least initially. Research training and research projects require careful planning in order to be successful.

Chapter 3

An overview of how to approach research tasks

Solitary, meditative observation is the first step in the poetry of research, in the formation of scientific fantasies, the reality of which we then test with the tools of logic, mathematics, physics and chemistry.

Theodor Billroth 1829–94

From an idea to a plan

Success in research, and in research degrees programmes, requires careful planning. While success may be measured in terms of a research project that attracts a research grant, is completed on time and within resources, is reported in both a major thesis of 40–80 000 words and papers published in peer-reviewed journals, and perhaps influences decision making, achieving this is no accident. In many ways a research project requires the same planning approach as major building projects, devising the plan, considering what resources are necessary, when the resources are available, and then arranging for everything to happen as planned. Further, there should be back up plans to manage the almost inevitable changes that will have to be made in response to unexpected incidents or results. For health professionals, the added complications of work and personal lives have to be accommodated.

There are several issues to consider in planning a successful research project, and these are listed in Box 3.1. The rest of this chapter briefly discusses each of these tips, and subsequent chapters explore some of the issues in greater depth.

Choosing the research topic and question

All early researchers begin with research questions that are too big, perhaps big enough for several PhDs and with possible answers that would merit a prize,

---

Box 3.1 Tips for successful navigation of a research programme.

- Choose a research topic that is personally interesting
- Look around for a supervisor with the time, interest and expertise to support the research
- Cut initial over-ambitious ideas down to an answerable question
- Focus early on literature reviews and methodology
- Estimate the resources (time and money) that are available to support the project
- Identify and apply for funds to support the project
- Address potential ethical issues and obtain ethics approval
- Plan journal publications as you write the main thesis

but in reality research training is less about making *the* discovery and more about learning how to conduct sound research. Therefore research projects should be trimmed to become manageable tasks that allow for acquisition of research skills within an achievable project.[1]

One advantage that more mature and experienced research students have is that they can choose a research topic that is of personal interest, usually because it arises from their professional practice experience and is therefore relevant to their future practice. By comparison, many younger research students simply join an experienced team and have little or no choice over their research topic, although of course can still acquire research skills, even if the research topic is not particularly interesting. However, with the slower time frame of professional research students, it is wise to have a positive 'relationship' with the research topic, as students may have to live with their research project for quite a long time.

Matching research students and supervisors

The relationship between student and supervisor is of extreme importance. One of the commonest reasons for students withdrawing from research degrees is a break in the relationship. Such a break may be due to one of several things: the supervisor moves to another university, becomes ill, dies or retires; or the student-supervisor relationship is dysfunctional. The traditional research student model involved a close apprenticeship between the student and usually one experienced researcher, and this is the most fragile model, because it depends on having a functional one-to-one relationship that lasts the entire period of enrolment, during which there may well be pressures around ideas, resources, timelines and other issues. It is therefore essential for students and supervisors to select each other carefully.

Trimming ideas to achievable projects

It is common for novice researchers to want to answer a question of earth-shattering importance, and very unlikely that even the most successful PhD project will go anywhere near that level of achievement. Being immersed in professional practice brings both the advantage of relevance and the disadvantage of potential complexity, as issues encountered in professional practice are more likely to be entangled in the 'messy' real world, where it can be very difficult to 'unbundle' associations and cause/effect relationships. While it is appropriate to commence with a broad research 'area' of interest, early advice is helpful to trim this to a clearer, simpler research question that will provide an appropriate platform for research training.[2] The 'action research' model is one way of linking research methods to professional practices.[3]

Start by building on previous research achievements

Individual research projects rarely make a quantum leap in knowledge and understanding, but instead build incrementally on the achievements of earlier research. If, as they should, those achievements have been documented in accessible academic literature, then a key early task is to seek that literature.[4]

This will help with both the task of refining research questions to achievable projects and the task of exploring potential research methods. When reading the literature, pay special attention to the methods section, as learning research methodology is one of the main aims of any research degrees. Further, under-taking a research degree requires a research method that is appropriate to the research question, and the literature is where the application of research methods is documented. Failure to adopt or apply the most appropriate method can ruin projects starting with the cleverest of ideas, if they produce either the wrong or incorrectly interpreted data.

Time and other resources

Research projects do not happen by accident, in spare time or for free. High quality research is expensive, takes time and requires planning. Just how much funding, time and other resources are necessary will depend on the nature of the research question and the methods chosen. It is often assumed that the time of research students comes for free or little cost and is permanently available, but that is not the case for professionals taking time out of practice to conduct research. Professional practice has to be provided and, in combination with family and other personal commitments, reduces both time availability and the income of research students. While there are often no easy options and progress is necessarily slower, research students taking time out from practice need to plan how their professional practice time will be replaced. The key point is that the resources needed to support the research project need to be identified early. This is both part of research training and a necessary step to ensure that the project is achieved. The choice of methods will heavily influence the resource requirements, and must be determined before a resource plan can be finalised. Good results can be achieved on tight budgets, and it is better to plan a project to the available resources rather than have to curtail projects through lack of funding.

Identifying and applying for funding

Once resource requirements are determined, potential researchers should explore all possible funding opportunities, including scholarships and research grants that might make easier the transition to student life and fund more adventurous data gathering. There are many possible avenues for research funding, both internal and external to universities, and going through the exercise of writing a proposal for research funding is an important skill that should be learned by research students, particularly at doctoral level. These sources include: national priority-led research pools (e.g. Medical Research Council); charities (e.g. a national cancer research fund); a wide range of independent, named, bequest-based funding schemes; research support schemes managed by professional organisations (e.g. Royal Colleges); and research-priming schemes within most universities. Each of these schemes will have clearly described aims, objectives, priorities, application forms and application processes. Such information is widely accessible via relevant web sites, and they are easily identifiable through any reasonable web search engine. The graduate research offices within all universities will have information on both their own internal schemes and external schemes. Potential supervisors should also be able to provide guidance, aided by their particular content expertise and experience applying for funding. One option that is more available to researchers with questions that are highly applicable to the workplace is to approach employers in health care, as they may be willing to make a contribution through either paid release from duties or direct research funding, in expectation of a benefit to the workplace in return for the investment. A further option for projects relevant to health professional practice is to apply through the relevant professional organisation for a research grant, a research training fellowship or both.

Depending on the success of applications for support, the size or scope of the research may have to be trimmed; this means that research students might have to have a 'Plan A/Plan B' approach, with two research plans, reflecting both the desired and actual resource availability.

Consider ethical issues and obtain ethics approval

Research ethics is now a complex set of issues that require careful consideration before research can proceed. Research ethics committees typically include membership from a wide range of groups in order to ensure that the many possible perspectives are incorporated and that the research will not cause harm to any individuals or society. Further, where animals are involved, they must be treated humanely. Even at the level of student research projects, research always has the potential to cause harm, even if unintentionally, and risks must be predicted, considered and where possible avoided.

For research projects involving health professionals, animal involvement is unlikely. If it is to be included, there are very detailed and specific requirements that must be adhered to. These are available through the university graduate research office, but also widely available via government department websites. It is more common for health research to involve patients, another complex area that has detailed and specific requirements, again available from the graduate research office or government/health sector websites. Two key issues are informed consent and patient confidentiality. All research projects have to ensure that data is collected only with very clear, written consent of patients and the health care system managers, and that collected data cannot identify participating patients. A third issue that is commonly encountered in educational research is the power imbalance between learners and teachers. Teachers cannot expect, require or coerce learners into participating in research. Instead, they must ask nicely after complete explanation of the project and proceed only with formal written consent. Results of research, and decisions about whether or not to participate in the research, must not have any role in academic progress decisions. Again, students should seek advice from their supervisors and the graduate research office.

Plan research journal publications

Unpalatable as it may sound to some, a significant measure of success of research degrees is the publication of research findings in appropriate academic journals. This is part of research training, but its main importance is that it closes the loop, as it is the academic way of reporting results back to the literature that informed the research. It is wise to think early about what publishable papers might come out of a research project – experienced researchers can do this – and to plan the publications early as part of the process of writing both the thesis and any journal papers simultaneously. While these are different tasks that require different approaches, there is synergy in doing both at the same time.[5] Academic writing is an important issue in its own right, and it is wise to seek advice early about how to write for an academic or scientific audience.[6]

The structure of research degrees

One of the least understood aspects of a research degree programme is its structure. There are formal requirements and rules for enrolment periods, confirmation seminars, periodic progress reports, exit seminars, and thesis submission; these are the internal signposts that guide research students and supervisors. While there are generic requirements, such as period of candidature, the need to produce a thesis, academic writing style etc., there are also degree level specific and institution specific requirements. These include variations in admission requirements, pre-requisite academic achievement, steps in the research project supervision, word length of theses, alternatives to theses, and theses marking processes. This level of detail cannot be provided in a small book like this, so readers should be familiar with the requirements of *their* degree in *their* university.

The rules are usually written for full-time students rather than for professionals juggling part-time research, clinical practice and family demands. The former are more likely to be attached to a successful research team and work to the established routine of that team, often on part of a larger project. This means that timelines almost define themselves, as the research team works both in parallel and together towards a completion of a research plan.

On the other hand, more mature, part-time research students are more likely to be following a more independent path, with their own research questions and more complex lives. This means that their research projects follow a less linear path. However, all research projects have in common an overall structure and process into which most research students can fit.

The first of these concerns the approximate proportion of time that research students should devote to certain components of the research project process. In broad terms there are three phases to a research student project. The first is the 'getting ready to gather data/information' phase, which is all about refining ideas, reading the literature, selecting the appropriate methods, and ensuring the necessary resources are available. The second phase is where the data or information is gathered. The third phase is the data analysis/interpretation and reporting/writing phase. These three phases can overlap, but it is useful for novice researchers to consider following the model more closely.

Figure 3.1 presents in diagram form this generic structure for a research degree. The *x*-axis is the timeline, which for PhD programmes could be up to eight years part-time. The *y*-axis indicates the probable variation in academic scope of the project, and the dotted lines represent the probable expansion of knowledge over time. The timeline is divided approximately into thirds, with the first third of enrolment (a) comprising reading around an initially broad research area,[4] a narrowing down to (b) a more specific and manageable

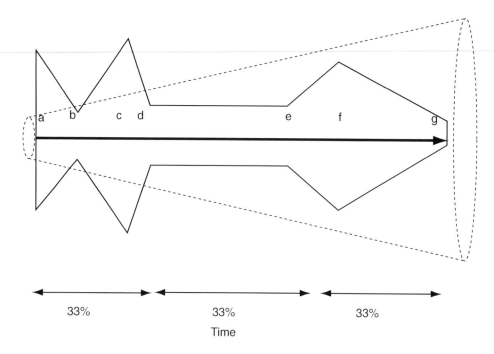

Figure 3.1 Scope and knowledge acquisition in a research programme.

research topic, and then (c) reading more broadly around the methods required for that topic, before (d) completing the research design and plan.

The middle third, from (d) to (e), is where the student focuses on gathering the data or information according to the research plan. During the final third of time, on completion of information gathering, students then (f) broaden the scope as they consider the findings and link them to the literature, before (g) focusing on writing the final report. Meanwhile the breadth of knowledge (dotted lines) of the student should increase throughout the project, as the reading of the literature throughout should expose them to a wider range of issues than covered in the narrower project. While this is a highly idealised model of the apparent tension between breadth of learning and focus on a narrow research topic during a research degree, it fits with the author's experiences as both a student and a supervisor.

The key phase is the first. If the research question is not clear, achievable and linked to the literature, if the wrong methods are chosen and if the resources are not secured, the next two phases can be very messy and the result will likely be poor.

Another tool for planning a research project is to borrow a generic project management tool – a wall chart that can be hung in front of your desk as a reminder. This is a visual representation of timelines, and sequences that, if followed, allow for efficient progress to be made on time and on budget. Key deadlines are clearly indicated, and regular team meetings keep all components of the project on track. Project charts are commonly used in a wide variety of projects, particularly construction and industrial projects. They help project

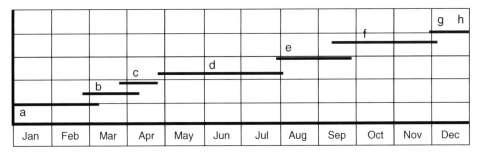

a = literature review
b = refining research questions
c = determining research methods
d = gathering data/information

e = data analysis
f = report writing
g = finalising report/catch up
h = party!

Figure 3.2 Research project chart plan.

managers with very simple, yet essential issues such as when to order 100 trucks of concrete or to call in the electricians, plumbers and roof builders.

A simple example of a project chart for a research project is provided in Figure 3.2, which indicates graphically the approximate timing and sequencing of a research project plan that should be completed within 12 months. Note that many individual tasks overlap, as it is necessary to multi-task at times. It is wise to build in predicted periods of inactivity, such as a planned vacation, and also to leave time towards the end to allow catching up or re-writes of the report.

Project charts are not the only way of displaying the relevant information. Another is a more simple form of timeline-activity description, an example of which is in Table 3.1. This example would represent a relatively small project that was manageable within an academic year. The plan however has a major flaw.

The serious flaw in the example project plan in Table 3.1 is that it suggests that data will be collected in December to February. This is extremely optimistic, as at that time of year people are often not particularly interested in data collection, because of vacations, the weather or some other reason. Elections, wars and major public debates can be good for some kinds of research, but distracting for others. There are several key times when research progress may be affected, including all vacation periods, public holidays etc. While these periods may be appropriate (perhaps even ideal) for thinking, reading the literature and writing reports, data collection may be severely constrained. It is wise to build

Table 3.1 Example project timeline sheet.

Project activity	Timeline
Literature review	September–October
Select methods	November
Collect data	December–February
Analyse data	March
Write report	April–June

research plans around predicted periods of difficulty, and to build in flexibility to deal with unexpected situations.

Project timeline charts will not by themselves keep projects on target, but if realistically constructed and followed, can improve project management and help organise the less experienced researchers. They are not necessarily popular with researchers, many of whom operate at a more intuitive level that is based on experience. However, novice researchers may find them very helpful, particularly when approaching a slower, part-time research degree that has to allow for work and personal/family time. On the other hand, novice researchers will be less experienced at constructing the charts, and supervisors should offer their experience to their students in helping them develop an achievable project plan. This may be particularly helpful for the slower, longer term project trajectories of health professionals in part-time research training programmes. More experienced researchers are better at developing project charts, as they will have a more realistic idea of how long each phase or component should take, so novice researchers should seek advice. For example, one of the commonest errors novice researchers make is knowing when to stop searching the literature and finalise research questions and methods. This is because the answers may not be there, and this research project may be genuinely building on a current gap in the literature. The judgment about when to say 'enough is enough' and get on with data/information gathering is a difficult one for novice researchers. There should be meetings between research students and their supervisors around the times that such judgements have to be made.

Case studies
Case A

Jamie has made some progress, in that the course director has found a colleague – the Director of Medical Education – in the medical education office, who is interested in Jamie's question. This colleague meets with Jamie and appears to provide conflicting advice. On the one hand, she says that the question is fascinating and lots of educators have similar thoughts, so any progress that Jamie might make would probably be of broad interest. On the other hand, she says that she is not sure exactly what Jamie's question is, as it is just too broad. She advises Jamie to look at the literature and see what research might have been done in the general area. This might help him refine his ideas to a more specific and manageable research question. She also advises Jamie to enrol in some research training modules in both quantitative and qualitative methods, but he is reluctant to do that as he is not really interested in doing more than a simple project. Jamie finds all this a bit frustrating.

Case B

Ahmed is advised that there are a couple of people with some interest in the general area of patient pathways, but that they are not in the School of Nursing. Ahmed is directed to an academic in the School of Management at another, nearby university. The meeting goes well, as this academic is quite passionate about the general topic, although is not a health professional and has no professional content knowledge at all. Rather to Ahmed's surprise, he says that his lack of content expertise is not important and he offers to help supervise a research project that might fit into the masters course that builds on Ahmed's current postgraduate diploma course. The research methods components of that course are providing a broad appreciation of research methodology, and Ahmed finds that he can have an understandable discussion about the differences required for his project.

Case C

Susan discovers in her reading that there is an academic speech therapist at another university who appears to share her interests and has done some research around validation and benchmarking of tests in collaboration with an educational psychologist. She makes contact, initially by email, and then by phone, and the discussions are very interesting. There is a gap here in both the literature and in clinical practice, and therefore scope to make a genuine contribution. It is soon clear that these three people may be able to embark on a doctoral level research project, based on Susan's question. Susan is keen, and the discussion moves on to how to do that.

Conclusion

Good research, and good research training, requires careful planning and progress through semi-discrete phases of a research project. This chapter has taken an overview of the structure and process of research projects, with an emphasis on the more professionally relevant projects, and has proposed both a model of progress to follow and a project management tool to help novice researchers stay on track. Subsequent chapters will explore in greater depth some of the key issues in ensuring a successful research degree outcome.

References

1   Hays RB. Research in general practice: getting started. *Australian Family Physician*. 1991; **20**: 1751–3.

2   Kelly G. Action oriented research. *Australian Family Physician*. 2000; **29**: 711–12.

3   Underwood P, Murray S. Defining the question. *Australian Family Physician.* 1998; **27**: 173–5.

4   Wilson I. Searching the literature. A beginner's guide. *Australian Family Physician*. 1998; **27**: 385–6.

5   Hays RB. Publishing Pointers. *Australian Family Physician*. 1996; **25**: S11–S14.

6   Peat JK, Elliot EJ, Baur LJ, *et al. Scientific writing: Easy when you know how*. London: BMJ Books, 2002.

Chapter 4

Refining research themes and topics

The object of research is the advancement not of the investigator, but of knowledge.

Mervyn H Gordon 1872–1953

Research triggers

The ideas for research typically emerge from reflection on issues encountered in professional practice. It is quite common for professionals to come up against patients or clients that do not fit the rather classical frameworks that form the basis of the curricula they studied during training. While these frameworks are useful tools at the commencement of professional life, they were not really designed to cover all possible issues of diagnosis or management. Even in an era of evidence-based health care, there is still a substantial proportion of professional practice for which there is no, little or conflicting research evidence. Experience is what individuals use to work out what to do when there is insufficient evidence to guide practice and provide the best care possible.

This is a steep learning experience, particularly during the early years of practice. Roughly speaking, there are two positive outcomes. The first is that individuals usually develop into competent professionals with an appropriate blend of theoretical knowledge and practical experience, and ideally maintain that over many years as knowledge and practice evolve. The second is that those gaps or mismatches between learned frameworks and real practice may trigger a desire to find out why there is a mismatch or gap, and what can be done about it.

Hence health professionals considering doing research generally have a strongly applied approach – driven by current practice, building on previous evidence, and shaping future practice. This kind of research often does not attract the same level of formal academic recognition, funding or other support as does biomedical laboratory research, but is no less important in the advancement of health care. Indeed, it is often the kind of research that most directly affects the healthcare experience of patients.

However, it is usual for the questions that arise from practice to be rather broad. One example is that of our first case study in which Jamie wants to explore why some learners achieve better than others. While this is a laudable ambition, there are many factors which could explain variations in learning achievement. Such questions are too large to be answered in a research training project, because they comprise several small components that need to be addressed, and not necessarily at the same time. Questions emerging from professional practice often have to be de-constructed into bite-sized chunks that are answerable. Following Jamie's example further, the broad question has to be narrowed by choosing a more precise learning activity in a particular context, such as consultation skills in junior registrars.

Identifying research themes

A research trigger is just that – the germ of an idea – and it needs to be nurtured and developed as it becomes a clearer research question that is worth answering. Sometimes a trigger is not worth developing, generally for one of three possible reasons. The first is that it remains too vague to be meaningful. For instance, should Jamie not be able to get beyond his relatively broad and vague research trigger and develop something that is clear and achievable, then he will not get far. Second, in the search for other information to help clarify the question, it may be found that someone else has answered the question, but you had not heard about it. This is a common situation, as knowledge advances fast and no individual can be familiar with current debate in every relevant research journal, although the narrower the speciality, the easier it becomes to keep abreast of the contents of a few journals. All professionals should try hard to access recent developments in the literature, even by one of the more accessible abstracting services. The third reason is that answering the question is beyond the resources of the individual who thought of the trigger. For example, again following Jamie's case, there may be influences on learning outside the control of an individual teacher, health facility or even training institution. Jamie needs to focus on what he can influence, and one outcome of his research may be identification of factors that should be addressed by other stakeholders, such as the health facility, the training institution or society in general (the latter is really difficult!). Those stakeholders may be better placed and better resourced to pursue important issues of relevance to them.

The next step is to stand back from the trigger, read the literature, discuss the ideas with others, and try to see what the research question is. As part of this thinking, it is often wise to identify research themes, as this is generally how the literature (key words and phrases), researchers and other resources, and research methods are organised. More specific literature and advice will be accessed if the conversation is about probable themes than the original question, even if the first attempt at identifying themes does not capture the essence completely. This step can be deferred until a discussion with a researcher, but the discussion will not get far until themes are identified. As a rule, experienced researchers will be more adept at this stage, particularly if they are used to supporting novice researchers. Research themes may be either broader or more specific than the original triggers, but they make the forming of clear research questions easier. Table 4.1 lists some examples of research triggers, including those in our three case studies, and the research themes that match them.

Research themes to questions

Research themes are still generally too broad to be specific research questions, and in fact may lead to several possible research questions for each theme. This 'deconstruction' of themes to questions is often very helpful to novice researchers, as they can see why the original trigger appeared to be broad and unachievable. For example, the theme of patient access to health care resources raises several possible questions that are relevant to the original trigger. Is there a problem? Why is there a problem? What is the impact of the problem? What are the possible solutions to these problems? Do these solutions work? The situation is similar for other research triggers, although the simpler 'what works

Table 4.1 Research triggers to research themes.

Research triggers	Research themes
1 Some patients appear not to attend distant Oncology services.	1 Patient access to Oncology services.
2 Library reports that students in some courses hardly ever borrow books.	2 Student access and use of learning resources.
3 Patients respond differently according to treatment option.	3 Efficacy of treatment options.
4 Some learning activities do not work well.	4 Learning styles and methods.
5 Can minor injuries be managed more efficiently?	5 Efficiency and outcome of patient flows.
6 Developing or adapting language tests for certain population groups.	6 Validation for population groups.

Table 4.2 Research themes to research questions.

Research themes	Research questions
1 Patient access to Oncology services.	1 Do different groups access services differently? If so, why? Do different groups have different survival rates? What are the possible solutions? Do any of these work?
2 Student access and use of learning resources.	2 Do different groups access resources differently? If so, why? Are there differences in assessment results?
3 Efficacy of treatment options.	3 Is treatment A better than treatment B or placebo?
4 Learning styles and methods.	4 What are the components of the learning interaction? What do students think of them? Are there preferred activities? What effect does each have on learning?
5 Efficiency and outcome of patient flows.	5 What patient flow systems are possible? What are the potential advantages and disadvantages of each? Does one work better than others? What about cost-efficiency? Are there differences in patient outcomes?
6 Validation for population groups.	6 What are the different population groups? Should they have different norms and benchmarks? If so, why? What are the norms and benchmarks for each group?

best' theme is often simpler and clearer from the beginning. Table 4.2 lists the same themes from Table 4.1 and some possible research questions that flow from them.

Types of questions and the impact on research methods

So far readers may be assuming that there is always a clear research question to answer and a clear way of doing that. However, this is an over-simplification of the rather complex debate in research about what a research question should look like and whether or not one is even needed. This debate reflects the diversity of both what is called research and the methods that are used.

Just as practice produces the research questions, the question determines the research methods that are most appropriate to 'answer' the question. The dominant research paradigm in health care is quantitative research, where the aim is to answer questions, based on numbers of cases in both 'intervention' and 'control' groups. Ideally, the difference between groups (to which cases are randomly allocated) is just a single variable (the 'intervention'), a statistically significant difference in outcome is found, and the result can be extrapolated to other individuals who are similar to those in the intervention group. The key question is 'what is better', and the research question is usually re-framed as a hypothesis that is either confirmed or refuted by the research. For example, the research question 'is treatment A better than treatment B?' becomes the hypothesis 'patients treated with A will have a better outcome than those treated with B'. This kind of research aspires to be the classical research design that includes random group allocation, double blind, crossover design, a clear intervention in one group that is not applied in a 'control' group, the required numbers in each group, and statistical methods are used to process 'data' to demonstrate that the intervention is either better or not. This is the form of research most likely to be encountered in health professional schools, as it clearly contributes to progress in improving decisions about investigations and treatments.

However there is another research paradigm that can make important contributions to health care. This is qualitative research, which aims to improve understanding rather than answer questions. The key questions here are 'how' and 'why', the approach more 'inductive' than 'reductionist'. Statistical methods are not used, but instead 'information' derived from interviews and questionnaires is analysed by a variety of tools to generate lists of issues (themes) and perhaps consensus around those issues. This kind or research is increasingly important in understanding how, why and when patients behave and respond (or not) as they experience health care. More detailed information about research methodology can be found in many books and courses; this brief book should not be seen as a replacement for formal research methodology training!

While methodologists often fall into groups that use either quantitative or qualitative methods, and according to legend neither understand nor value the other paradigm, both methods are important and they are often combined to answer complex questions: the key issue is the nature of the question. An example is research that aims to explore the most effective treatment regime for a form of cancer. While quantitative methods will better determine if the intervention produces better survival rates than either no or another intervention, qualitative methods will better explore how patients feel about the treat-

Table 4.3 Comparison of quantitative and qualitative research.

Quantitative research	Qualitative research
Aims to answer precise questions	Aim to increase understanding
Requires numbers of patients in groups	Numbers less important
Participants and judges 'blind'	No blinding
Group allocation ideally random	Sampling reflects context
Statistical significance indicates success	Statistics not used
Results extrapolated to others	Results cannot be extrapolated

ment. What is the use of a new drug regime if it extends life by a few months but makes people feel so awful that they will not try it? Here the key wording in the research question is 'most effective', as effectiveness can include more than one measure and cover both quantity and quality of life. More complex questions often arise in primary care and medical education, the former because of greater uncertainty of diagnoses and increased difficulty controlling single interventions, and in the latter because of greater complexity of interventions and difficulty organising control groups. The differences between quantitative and qualitative methods are summarised briefly in Table 4.3.

Back to the kind of research question that might arise from professional practice. The question may be able to be framed as a question that required quantitative methods to provide an 'answer' about 'what is better'. This is most common with questions about 'intervention' such as investigations and treatments, where the answer will be option A, B, C etc., or perhaps none. On the other hand, the question may be about 'why', 'when' or 'how'. If so, then quali-

Table 4.4 Examples of questions that may arise according to research methods.

Research question	Primary research method
Which treatment modality is better?	Quantitative
Which investigation is the more accurate?	Quantitative
Why do patients access oncology services differently?	Qualitative
Why do students access certain learning resources?	Qualitative
What are the pros and cons of different patient pathways?	Qualitative
What pathway more efficiently manages minor trauma?	Quantitative
What does the profession think about current benchmarks for language tests in different populations?	Qualitative
What are the benchmarks for language tests with different populations?	Quantitative

tative measures are the most appropriate to explore perceptions, perhaps from different perspectives, and see if there are identifiable themes. In this kind of research the answer is likely to be an explanation, not a one-word answer. There is an analogy to communication skills in health care consultations, which health professionals will have been taught formally at some stage. There are close-ended questions, which seek to narrow and focus conversation through yes/no answers, and there are open-ended questions, which expand conversation and improve mutual understanding. Some examples of research questions are provided in Table 4.4.

Case studies

Case A

Jamie's question is a good example of a question that is applied to practice, yet is rather broad. While its origin is understandable, it is almost unanswerable without exploring several aspects, such as: what Jamie knows and does; the prior knowledge, skills and attitudes of each learner; the particular topic being discussed etc. There are several possible combinations of circumstances, each of which might be a unique situation and might have a unique set of reasons for certain outcomes. Jamie will have to learn that education can be quite 'messy' – there may be no such thing as a 'simple' question in education research – and he will have to develop a much clearer idea of just what he could do to contribute to answering his 'big' question. He is likely to need a combination of quantitative and qualitative methods, although he will need to refine the question further before being able to decide on that. He is still confident that things will work out, because he has some research experience from his undergraduate medical course. He is also not too concerned about resources for the moment, as he believes that direct costs will be low, at least until he has a clearer idea of what he will do. Arguably his greatest cost will be in personal effort, and he is confident that he can negotiate flexibility in his practice roster to allow him the necessary time to devote to the project. He has heard that the Royal College of General Practitioners and the Society for Academic Primary Care, both of which he is a member, have research grant schemes and part-time research training fellowships. Further, the head of the regional school of primary care education has hinted that there may also be support available from their funds, so long as the project addresses something of importance to postgraduate GP training.

Case B

Ahmed has a more circumscribed question that clearly combines issues of clinical judgement in triaging and treatment with decision flow issues. He is likely to need mainly quantitative methods and perhaps specific information technology and computer software support. However, he may not yet know this and his is still a relatively complex question that needs some refining before he can make progress. He is not sure about resource needs but will think about that when he has a clearer idea of what he will do, as he has heard that there may be funds available through the College of Nursing. He is willing to accept all advice as he recognises his inexperience in research.

Case C

Susan's question is the clearest and most specific. This should not be a surprise, as Susan has done some research training in addition to her professional practice experience. Therefore she has used those skills to achieve a position quite close to the point where she could commence research. Her project will use mostly quantitative methods, particularly a branch known as psychometrics (measuring behaviours), as she will have to gain sufficient data from her target population groups to develop benchmark scores that may define normal test values for those populations. Her clinical supervisor is willing to consider releasing her time and possibly even contributing some direct costs, as the potential value of the research is recognised. Meanwhile, Susan is seeking other potential sources of funding through discussion with her colleagues and professional contact, including the College of Speech Language Therapists.

Conclusion

This chapter has taken the reader on a journey from thinking of the original research idea (trigger) to formulate a clearer, answerable research question. The nature of research questions is broad, as research is a diverse field of endeavour. There are appropriate research methods for most research questions, many of which are not the classical biomedical, quantitative research designs that many health professional students will have encountered. Quantitative methods are more appropriate to questions that need a focused, definitive answer, while qualitative methods are more appropriate for questions that open up discussions and improve understanding. Getting the research question right is a key step in developing a research project, as selection of supervisors, identifying the necessary facilities and resources, and choosing the research design and methods, all depend substantially on the research question to be addressed.

Chapter 5

Successful supervision

I believe that a research committee can do one useful thing and one only. It can find the workers best fitted to attack a particular problem, bring them together, give them the facilities they need, and leave them to get on with the work.

William Whiteman Carlton Topley 1886–1944

An important relationship

After choosing a life partner, choosing a research supervisor is quite high on the list of high stakes relationships that occur in life's journey. It may be easier to end this relationship than a marriage, but if the relationship goes badly, both the stress levels and the chances of a poor academic result can be high.

The traditional model of research supervision involved an experienced, successful academic researcher with high content expertise. Students would vie for the services of these icons, as the research topics were generally highly relevant to the supervisor's expertise, and were therefore likely to be success- ful in both thesis marking and other academic communications, particularly as the supervisor could be very influential in selecting thesis markers, journals and conferences. In many respects the name of the supervisor on a cv meant more than having the research degree.

There are however problems with this model. When it works, it often works very well indeed, and has resulted in many high quality researchers coming through the ranks. However, if there are problems, the outcome can be terrible for both sides. Student-supervisor relationships are not made in heaven. What if the two just turn out to be the wrong chemistry of personalities? Some brilliant researchers can be rather idiosyncratic people with narrow expertise that might not include generic educational facilitation skills. Similarly, some students can be 'difficult' people. What if there are disagreements between supervisor and student? What if the supervisor does not understand the more complex life/work/study balance of part-time professional students? Who 'owns' the intellectual property (IP) of the project? Because of the power imbalance inherent in a student-teacher relationship, the supervisor almost always wins arguments and dominates discussions and direction. What if the supervisor leaves for another university, retires, becomes ill or dies? If that supervisor is no longer available, then the 'corporate memory' of the research project may also be unavailable.

The current approach in most universities is to focus on the provision of whatever support is necessary, rather than on individual research supervisors. It is unlikely that any individual could alone provide all of the required super- vision and support roles to minimise the chances of a poor outcome, whereas a team of supervisors should be able to do so. While the team approach offers remedies for most potential problems, care still needs to be taken in matching students to supervisors.

What kind of support is needed?

The larger the research project and the higher the level, the more important it is to have access to the widest range of expertise and support, and effective relationships with those providing the expertise and support. Three broad kinds of supervisory support are required for a student research project. The first is expertise in the content of the research project, including the ideas, current research status and relevant methodology. This expertise is more likely to be found in current, successful researchers. Second, expertise is required in the educational process of research supervision, including resources, timelines, institutional requirements for presentations and reports. This rather unselfish expertise may well be found in an experienced researcher who is content with their research success and now wants to focus on helping others start a similar journey. Third, expertise is required in supporting research students, including approachability, interest, flexibility, and negotiating skills. This is the person who can help sort out the inevitable problems that arise, often acting as the 'honest broker' with other supervisors and the institution. All of these skill sets are necessary. An ideal research supervision panel may be 2–4 individuals, each of whom contributes in a complementary manner.

Content expertise

Content expertise is the most obvious skill set that both students and supervisors consider, and is the main feature of the traditional approach. It is somewhat obvious that students who want to do well will seek out a supervisor who knows a lot about their intended research topic, as content expertise may be an advantage in accessing relevant literature and financial resources, as well as increasing the chances of a positive result that will be successfully reported in an academic outlet. From the perspective of successful researchers, it is attractive to have research students to add to a research team, as research students projects can add resources, strengthen teams working on their main research theme, or broaden research activity to topics related to their main theme.

It is important to recognise that a single content expert may not be sufficient. Depending on the nature of the research project, it may be wise to recruit additional supervisors with specific expertise, particularly around specific research methods. Depending on the question to be addressed, this may be more than one person. For example, projects requiring both quantitative and qualitative methods may well benefit from having two such supervisors, reflecting expertise in each research paradigms. Caution is required here, as sometimes the ideology of separate research paradigms interferes with the pragmatism of trying to answer a complex question through an eclectic combination of methods. Where possible, try to find a supervisor who is comfortable with the combination of methods you may need for the particular research question. Also, professionally relevant research projects often need the injection of different perspectives and expertise, as they often bridge 'professional' and 'academic' concepts and methods. For example, a health professional may benefit from having as a supervisor someone from within his or her own profession, as well as a supervisor who contributes specific research methodology expertise that is used across many professional or other contexts.

However, not all excellent researchers have an understanding of the research candidature requirements or strong interpersonal skills. Where a content expert does have one or both of these additional skill sets, he or she is likely to be a strong supervisor. Where such skills are weaker, then there is still potential for a strong and effective student supervision team, so long as other members have complementary skills that in combination are closer to the 'ideal' supervision skill set.

Process expertise

Some of the most successful research supervisors may be weaker on content expertise, but strong on understanding the process of a research candidature. Excellent researchers can be so pre-occupied with doing what they do best – research – that they are not particularly interested in the rules and hurdles faced by research students. This kind of expertise is important, as research candidacy is generally time-limited and has to meet targets. For example, 6–8 years sounds like a long time for a part-time PhD candidacy, but when life is busy it can be easy to defer key activities to 'later', and then find the workload is too much. Most institutions try to avoid this by placing milestones in the student candidacy and support services to help students make it through. For example, there may be deadlines for initial proposals, literature reviews, coursework components, confirmation and exit seminars etc. There may also be internal or external grant schemes to support research students. Further, there may be complex requirements for formatting theses, and students should adopt such requirements from the beginning, rather than having to face tedious formatting revisions later. While research students should be self-directed enough to be aware of these requirements and to keep themselves on track, it is very helpful if one of the supervisors has a detailed understanding of these arrangements and can guide their students to explore making use of all available resources. A key element in the success of research degrees is organisation, and a well organised supervisor can reduce the stress levels around deadlines. Sometimes this role falls to a faculty member who is appointed to coordinate all research student activity with the relevant faculty or school. This person will work closely with the university's central student research office.

Personal support

The final skills set falls under the category of having a supervisor who is a nice, facilitatory person who genuinely wants his or her students to do well, and in time to perhaps even surpass their own expertise and reputation. These skills are similar to those interpersonal skills that make health professionals effective in their clinical work: active listening skills; being non-judgmental; ability to provide constructive feedback; focused on helping people make their own, informed decisions; and willing to negotiate changes in arrangements and timelines. This is the patient, understanding person who can help research students solve any problems or crises that arise. They can be literally the shoulder to cry on when things are tough, the cajoler who gets projects back on track, even in a modified form or, as a last resort, the person who arranges suspension or, in extreme circumstances, even cancellation of the candidacy if other parts of life have to take precedence. This is a set of professional skills that is usually present in combination with either the content expertise, the process expertise, or both. However, it is possible for this to be completely absent: some successful researchers seem to have never faced problems in their career progress and just do not seem to understand or want to get involved if things go wrong. Therefore, while all research students should commence without expectation of rocky times, they should actively seek at least one supervisor who has the ability to help them through any problems that arise.

Supervision panels
Putting a supervision panel together

As already stated, the most common arrangement now is to have a panel of research supervisors, comprising individuals with a mix of skills that in combination should cover all of the above roles. As a rule, the graduate research office (the name may vary in different universities) will assist research students put a team together and make sure that all roles are included. Sometimes successful research teams come ready-made. That is, there may well exist teams of research supervisors with both the complementary roles and skills and a track record of success. Strong research teams often take their research training roles very seriously and strive to put together teams that will increase the chances of success, as success is in their own interests as much as the students'. There is often also a faculty- or school-based graduate research student advisor or manager, who coordinates research training closer to the research teams.

A common framework for research supervision panel selection is provided in Table 5.1. Please note that more than one role may be provided by a single supervisor, just as there may be additional members above the 'core'. A common addition is the head of the school or faculty, as this ensures that students are supported from the top of the organisational unit. Once this individual 'signs off' on the research student candidacy, it becomes the responsibility of the organisational unit to see that the project is supported, funded, managed and completed. This initiative has been introduced as a means of improving retention and completion rates, as it ensures that sound projects and research

Table 5.1 Research supervision panel membership: roles and individuals.

Roles	Core Yes/No	Most likely representative
Content expert 1	Y	Successful researcher
Content expert 2	Y	Successful researcher
Process expert	Y	Faculty/School research coordinator or research student monitor
Personal support	Y	Any of the above
Organisational authority	N	Faculty or School Head

students succeed. However, while the authority of the organisational unit confers these advantages, there are also constraints: only well thought through and planned research proposals are likely to achieve this higher level support.

Location of research supervisors

While there may be advantages in having the research panel located in the same institution and the same town/city, this can be quite constraining when tapping into necessary expertise, particularly for higher level (PhD) projects, where international excellence is more relevant. We live in an era of excellent information technology, and there is no reason why supervisors cannot be on the other side of the world, so long as they can make a contribution. Most institutions will require the primary supervisor to be an employee, but will be willing to include experts from elsewhere as associate supervisors for specific expertise. A geographically dispersed panel has to work differently, and the more distant supervisors will probably not attend meetings unless their travel plans bring them to town – that should of course trigger a full panel meeting. They can however contribute a lot via email, phone and even videoconference, although usually around very specific issues. The best way to use the distant supervisors may be to ask them questions to which they can respond, and later ask them to review drafts. A key issue is to develop a student-supervisor relationship that can make this arrangement work. In many ways, location is becoming much less relevant.

Multi-professional research panels

It is worth re-stating that the individuals who become part of the research panel should reflect the necessary expertise to increase the chances of a successful outcome. Supervisors are an important resource and this choice should be made carefully. Particularly with applied health care and educational practice research projects, the questions and concepts are often complex and cross traditional uni-professional lines. For example, health care education is a combination of health care practice, educational psychology, and sometimes health sociology. Patient flow research combines health care practice with management and sometimes econometrics. Validation of a language test combines health care practice, educational and cognitive psychology and linguistics. All may need qualitative and quantitative methodological expertise.

This multi-professional approach to research is the currently preferred, and almost certainly the correct, approach. Professional and research paradigms should not be seen as rigid or mutually exclusive areas, and research should eclectically choose the required resources as fits the question. The future often requires 'thinking outside of the square'.

This approach is however not uniformly accepted, as it actually challenges some supervisors who are used to working within narrower, more familiar and more comfortable territory. While many researchers find this challenge enjoyable, others may prefer not to participate, but rather focus on being very good in a narrow field, and that is no bad thing. Potential research students may also note raised eyebrows from their colleagues, who may interpret (incorrectly) a multi-professional panel as an indication that the project may be less relevant to the particular professional territory. However, the opposite view is well worth considering. Research that brings together different groups of expertise and methodology, and produces results relevant to all of the groups often produces very interesting research degree graduates, who have demonstrated flexible, lateral thinking and mastery of merging professional boundary concepts. We live in an era where such boundary riders often end up in professional leadership positions. Research panels that produce such graduates can earn well deserved kudos and academic success.

Research panel leadership

Ideally, research supervision panels work well together in a collegial manner, with each member respected and valued for their contributions. Universities however require the team to have a formal leader, an individual who assumes primary responsibility for day-to-day research student progress. With a title such as 'principal supervisor' attached, this leadership is usually assumed by the primary academic content expert, as this is the individual with whom the research student will have most frequent contact. Not every academic may be a 'principal supervisor', as there are pre-requisites that may vary among universities, but are based on a combination of research success, research supervisor training and prior research student supervision success. It also almost certainly a requirement that the principal supervisor, and indeed most or all panel members, should have achieved the same level of research training as the student is enrolling. That is, all PhD student supervisors should have a PhD. This has a further advantage of ensuring that supervisors know what it is like to be a research student.

Research panel meetings

While research students should be encouraged to develop the appropriate degree of self-directedness, all research degree candidatures should include regular meetings with some or all members of the supervisor panel. The panel may get together as a complete team only occasionally, generally for required milestones and deadlines, but research students should maintain regular contact with all members. The most frequent meetings may be with the content experts, as these are the people who have most input to the research projects. Initially meetings should be arranged often – perhaps weekly – as concepts are discussed, literature is reviewed, ideas are formed, questions are formulated and narrowed, and tasks are identified and assigned. One of the most serious errors research students and supervisors can make is assuming that things are going well and not scheduling meetings (see Chapter 6). Yes, successful academic and professionals are busy, and research students are also busy, but it is not difficult to book diary entries well in advance. It is better to cancel an unnecessary meeting than to be unable to arrange at short notice one that is needed.

The other members of the panel should be available on an 'as needed' basis, particularly for specific issues. The process expert will provide specific advice on meeting the institutional requirements, such as booking seminars and sending reminders about reports. Should this be the formal faculty or school research student coordinator, the individual in that post will be required to initiate contact every so often to check that all is well. If problems arise that cannot be solved by the content expert supervisors, then students should initiate contact with either this person, or, where present, the research student monitor post. All members of the panel are appointed to professional roles and expect (and enjoy!) the contact and being able to help.

The 'professionalisation' of research supervision

As can be inferred from several comments so far, universities are becoming much more interventionist in research student supervision. Not long ago failure to complete a research degree programme was relatively common, and noted with momentary sadness by all except the student. Good researchers attracted a steady supply of applications to be research students, and hence those that withdrew were replaceable.

More recently, however, research student data has become part of the assessment of the performance by universities, faculties, schools and individual researchers. Research students are a source of income to universities, at a higher rate than for undergraduate students, and much of it sponsored by government and industry. As a means of fostering research, students rarely pay any fees. Therefore, student withdrawals from research training now mean a financial loss to universities and sponsors.

In response, university performance is measured, in part, by research student numbers and completions. Therefore universities now have organisational structures, usually called Graduate Research Offices (or similar), that track research student progress. These structures may have direct relationships with research students, and may have local contacts within faculties or schools to ensure that research students are cared for. They may also be the primary implementers of policies that govern eligibility to be a research supervisor, research supervisor training, research supervision panel function, research student support, identify the milestones that indicate progress, and manage the marking of theses.

Graduate research offices have two broad, related roles. The first is to ensure that eligible students commence a sound research project, with a sound research supervision panel. The second is to maximise the chances of completion. These roles mean a level of intervention, much of it behind the scenes, in academic life. If all works well, only able students, with achievable projects and all necessary financial and human resources, will commence research projects. These students will not only complete their projects, but will complete within time and within budget, and achieve their due academic rewards – degrees, conference presentations and published papers – thus achieving rewards (more students, prestige and funding) for the university. This is a good deal for all concerned!

The ideal research student

While much of this chapter has focused on the roles and responsibilities of supervisors, research students also have responsibilities, and no discussion of research supervision would be complete without including them.

Research training is not necessarily an easy time and should be done for the right reasons. Yes, there can be the thrill of the intellectual chase, the feeling that one is contributing to new knowledge and understanding, perhaps for the first time in the specific context of the research project. Yes, there is a reward of sorts at the end: a degree that denotes a level of basic or more advanced research competence. Yes, sometimes there are more tangible career rewards: promotion, new roles, higher income. However, most of the rewards are less tangible and involve a sense of personal satisfaction. People should embark on a research training pathway only if they are motivated primarily by gaining personal satisfaction. Never commence research training if the only goal is a promotion or increased income or status, as disappointment is the most likely outcome!

What can get in the way of success? Well, just about anything! Health professional research students are generally more mature, older, more applied, and potentially more distracted by competing personal and professional interests. They will have varied interests and personalities. Becoming a student again will almost certainly increase pressure, because workload is generally increasing and income often decreasing. Balancing personal and professional lives can be much more complex when there are two 'professional' roles (health worker and research student) than when balancing just one job and personal lives, even if the intended overall workload does not increase.

There will also be a change in status. In one part of work life the research student may be an experienced (even senior), confident professional, responsible for the supervision of others and able to make important decisions. In the other part of life this person is suddenly starting at the bottom of another pathway, inexperienced in research, less confident in their knowledge, and having to seek and accept advice from others. The locus of control shifts from more internal to more external, at least initially.

There may well be preferred learning styles that make research training more enjoyable and successful. There are many ways of looking at learning styles, but some attributes that may make research training more interesting and possible are an interest in theoretical knowledge and self-directedness. People who enjoy working out *why, how* and *what if,* rather than just *doing* or following guidelines, are probably more interested in understanding and contributing to theory. People who are capable of (and enjoy) making decisions about what best meets personal learning needs are probably more self-directed learners. More mature students may understand their preferred learning style better, but if not, the simple questionnaires referred to in Chapter 1 can be completed to increase self-awareness of learning styles.

Hence research students should make sure that they are both able and ready to commit to the rigours of devoting a substantial period of time to these changed circumstances – a potentially precarious balancing act – while allowing personal life to go on. This is a decision that has to be made by the individual research student, ideally after discussion with potential supervisors, other research students and employers. While some research projects may allow for breaks to be taken between stages, others are not easily broken down into component parts. Therefore, it may be wise to defer either starting the whole project, or the next stage of the project, if there is a predictable disruption to either personal or primary working lives. Work examples include upcoming transfer or promotion to new roles, events that are likely to distract from research training.

In some circumstances, the research project around which research training is built is of more direct benefit to the workplace. In such circumstances, the work environment may be made more flexible by understanding bosses who regard the results of the project as part of managing their organisational unit. An example might be a project about developing, implementing and evaluating a new way of providing clinical or educational service. Such a close connection between professional work and research training may be difficult to achieve, but demonstrates *par excellence* the closer relationship often seen in applied professional research.

Case studies

Case A

Jamie manages to fit in time to look around the literature, and to attend an international conference on medical education that this year happens to be not far away. At that meeting he hears presentations from several people whose papers he has read. This is a really interesting experience for Jamie, who sees just how passionate and sensible these people seem to be. He thinks through his potential research question over and over, and starts to see that what he is really interested in is how learners respond to feedback. This helps him focus his literature searches and discussions with researchers, including some of the presenters he enjoyed hearing at the conference. He finds the international medical education community to be very collegial and supportive, and decides to proceed with a modest research project, based on the material he has read and heard. He is worried about the amount of time this might take, as he has a very busy life as a clinician and an educator, and so although he can see how he could embark on a bigger project, he discusses with the director of medical education the possibility of being supervised in a research project that would make up most of the masters degree, rather than just a small component of it. They agree that it would be appropriate for him to ask for one of the current research leaders in the field, with whom he has been having email discussions, to join as a co-supervisor. He is also advised strongly to enrol in a module in research methods as part of his further development of the project. He is still not keen on this step but reluctantly agrees, as he has come to the realisation that education research is different to the small project he did as a student and that there may be no such thing as a 'simple and small' education research project.

Case B

Ahmed finds that his dual research supervision team, comprising people from very different perspectives – nursing and management – is working well. He finds the meetings with them enjoyable and their advice helpful. The Medical Director of the Emergency Department in which Ahmed works also offers assistance for specific clinical input, and even offers to approach her Royal College for funding support. To Ahmed's surprise he is awarded a small grant in return for presenting a paper on the results at a College conference. He accepts this as it will help with the purchase of some software. Some of his work colleagues are puzzled as they wonder if he is leaving clinical nursing, but Ahmed is pleased to get the multi-professional support.

Case C

Susan has several meetings with her two potential supervisors and gets on well with both of them. They seem to recognise and respect her passion for the task, and appear to be happy to help her achieve a mutually beneficial outcome. If all goes well, the supervisors will receive credit through the success of a project that may attract research funding, provide a contribution to both academic literature and profession practice, and lead to conference presentations and academic papers. For Susan, the reward will be a PhD and perhaps significant career development, but at the moment she is just having an enjoyable time!

Conclusion

Matching of research students to research supervisors is one of the most important early tasks in research training. These are key relationships that may have to withstand both easy and difficult times over a prolonged period of time, perhaps 6–8 years. Successful research supervision requires an almost super-human job description that is best managed by a panel of individuals who each contribute components such as content expertise, process expertise, student support expertise, and familiarity with the rules of the particular university. In return, potential research students must be able to devote considerable time and effort to their complex lives, balancing the demands of work, study and personal life. Increasingly, universities are investing resources in increasing the chances of successful research student outcomes.

Chapter 6

Surviving common pitfalls

It does happen exceptionally that a practising doctor makes a contribution to science...but it happens much oftener that he draws disastrous conclusions from his clinical experience because he has no conception of scientific method, and believes, like any rustic, that the handling of evidence and statistics needs no expertness.

George Bernard Shaw 1911

An interesting life

Whether or not the term 'an interesting life' is a curse is an interesting debate, and the life of a research student can encompass the full meaning of the phrase. As stated previously, one of the distinguishing features of health professionals who undertake research after a period of professional practice is that they are generally more mature, more experienced in life, more self-directed and amidst more complex personal and family circumstances. Many of these features make for very positive research experiences that can make a difference, but these may come at some personal cost. Careful planning can minimise the cost through establishing the appropriate and flexible supports at home and at work.

The day job

In an ideal world research training would be funded at professional practice incomes with as much time as necessary devoted to work, free from distractions, but it is not certain that such a world exists. For most professionals in research, professional practice continues at least part-time, as that is the main source of income that supports personal and family life and pays the mortgage etc. This means that health professional research students have to spend a substantial proportion of work time involved in patient care, rather than the pursuit of new knowledge, and be able to focus their energy and intellect to that important task. Occasionally a research student will receive formal support from work (income and released time) if their project is of immediate relevance to the workplace. This is an ideal situation, and all health professional students should consider the possibility of making their applied research project relevant to their workplace, not just for the likelihood of additional support, but also because it provides an immediate application of their research into professional practice. That can be very satisfying.

   While full-time research scholarships cannot provide the accustomed level of income, a balance of part-time practice and part-time research scholarship achieves the dual goals of quarantining research time and bringing in some income. It also formalises an arrangement that releases the research student from professional work. It is most unwise to spend that released time anywhere near the normal workplace, as it is equally important to devote research time to thinking about and conducting the research, free of distractions. Colleagues may not understand the boundary between professional and academic time and that peace and quiet is required for thinking ('headspace'), so it is better to do that thinking somewhere else.

The proportion of time spent on professional practice versus research training is a difficult one that is determined mostly by happenstance. However, beware agreeing to a 50/50 split of time. Most people with two 50% jobs find that they have two almost full-time jobs, as neither half is regarded as the primary role. It is therefore better to have a clear primary role, which takes precedent. This is most likely to be professional practice, and care must still be taken to protect the part-time research proportion. As a rule, clinical service delivery dominates health professional life, and in some jobs there will be a component of urgent or after-hours work to which the whole team, including the research student, must contribute. Research training also has an impact after hours, because it is often quieter and less hurried. This is when a lot of thinking can be done. While proportions can and should vary flexibly over the longer term, it is important (and difficult) to make sure that the flexibility is both ways.

The key to professional practice and research training proportions is sound planning, developing the skills to switch tasks, and negotiating clear agreements with employers and colleagues. Patience and a sense of humour are helpful personality traits. Ideally, any agreements should be in writing, as personnel can change and corporate memory can be lost. A written agreement might not solve all disputes that arise, but they at least prove that an agreement was made.

Family and friends

One's job can be a source of considerable stress for family relationships, and combining professional practice with research training may well increase those pressures. Neither professional practice nor research training (indeed any research) fits well into a nine-to-five, five day a week time-frame. Family members will therefore find their beloved research student likely to be distracted by one or other role at various times. Thoughts coincide at unpredictable times, and if an 'Aha' research moment occurs during dinner, the research student might dash off and make notes. Full-time researchers have notoriously flexible life styles, because they work at rather odd times, when the mood takes them. There is a form of creativity in research, rather like that of an artist, and to a certain extent work is motivated by inspiration. This can be difficult to live with!

Keeping family and friends on side is again largely down to choosing the right time of life and careful planning. Financial problems, the imminent birth of a child, responsibility (even shared) for three children under the age of four, or a terminally ill close relative provide really difficult challenges. It is not that one could not succeed in research training in such circumstances, but that it would be much more difficult. Even if there are no such difficulties, thinking ahead is wise to predict pressure points and plan flexible support for family responsibilities.

There are many reports of PhD students having serious relationship breakdowns. Just how much of this might be due to the research training is not known, but all intending research students should be aware of the potential for increased pressure on personal and family life, and do their best to prevent, predict and deal early with any problems. One of the research supervisor roles (see Chapter 5) is personal support and mentoring, and problems should be discussed with the person providing that role. All universities have student support and counselling services that may be able to help.

Personal issues

Research students, however mature and experienced, are people and therefore subject to the full range of human possibilities. That is they can become ill or have personal relationship problems. Should this happen, then it is almost certain that there will not be time to think about research and make progress. The student should seek advice from the research panel and student support service and consider the options. Depending on the stage of the research, it may be difficult to reduce the workload. Unless the problem is very short term, the wisest path may be to suspend the project and enrolment until things improve. It is better to focus energy on sorting out personal issues than to do poor research and fail to achieve the desired goals. Once things have improved, enrolment can resume.

Supervisors

Supervisors are generally committed academics, with strong personal interests around their areas of expertise and willingness to help their research students do well. However, within their academic roles they will vary in their research experience, research supervision experience, teaching skills and experience. Beyond their professional role, they are people too, and so face the normal human challenges of health and happiness.

Beyond individual supervisor characteristics, there is the chemistry of relationships between individuals. Supervisors in the panel have to get on with each other and work as a team, each respecting the others' roles and expertise. Supervisors should get on well with their students, with whom there has to be a relationship based on mutual respect and trust. Supervisors often find the supervision of more experienced professionals to be challenging, as the research student may well have considerable expertise in their professional life and indeed be the main source of inspiration for a research project arising from the student's professional context. The challenge for both supervisor and student is to recognise each other's expertise and work as a team.

Both kinds of relationships are professional roles that, if disrupted, can cause problems for research students. The onus for resolving such problems lies with the university, but experienced health professionals may well have some skills that can help with predicting and intervening early.

There are several kinds of possible disruptions. One is where a supervisor is offered a promotion to move elsewhere: career enhancement for academics often involves moving, sometimes internationally. This problem can often be managed quite easily as, if the student-supervisor relationship is sound, the support can continue over a distance. The nature of access to support will change to email and occasional face-to-face contact, but as discussed in Chapter 5, distance is no barrier to research supervision panel membership.

A more serious problem arises when a supervisor cannot continue any involvement, most likely through illness or even death. This is uncommon, but possible. Apart from the personal stress of losing contact with a person with whom there may be a strong relationship, from the narrower research perspective there may be difficulty in replacing the research or support expertise of the 'lost' supervisor. Other panel members will be in the best position to identify a replacement, although more advanced students at more advanced stages might have interacted with an appropriate person during the project, perhaps at a meeting or through the literature.

A related problem is where a supervisor has some form of personal crisis and, while still on the panel, does not contribute effectively. This can be quite destabilising, particularly if the supervisor's contribution is vital at the current stage of the research, and can be worse than having an absent supervisor. It is possible for a research student to be drawn into the supervisor's personal life problems, but this is extremely unadvisable. There is always a line between personal and professional lives that should not be crossed, and both students and supervisors should respect that line. If a research student feels that the relationship is becoming non-professional or unhelpful, they should seek advice from either another member of the panel or the research office.

Serious problems with supervisors are fortunately not common. Some conflict between supervisor panel members and between students and supervisors is almost inevitable and probably quite healthy, as research can be a dynamic process that combines the thrill of the chase with setbacks. The ideal research team works through these together, and students can learn a lot by being part of the process. However conflict can be very unpleasant, and unresolved conflict can lead to significant disruption to the research project and training. Both sides should try to resolve issues early. The student is by definition in the weaker position, but in this book we are discussing more experienced professional research students who should have more self-confidence and life skills. However, some problems may have to be resolved with external assistance.

It is also possible for research students and supervisors to just not be compatible people. This is a two-sided issue that probably comes down to personality clashes. If a supervisor suspects that he or she just cannot develop or maintain an effective supervisory relationship, he or she should initiate either a lesser role or withdrawal from the panel. If a student suspects a personality clash is developing, he or she should seek advice from other members of the panel or the research office. Early intervention on a 'no fault' basis is usually the best solution. Supervisors with a record of several personality clashes may well have a problem, but it is for the university to work that out. On the other hand, if a research student has several personality clashes (i.e. with the whole panel and with replacements), the problem is probably with the student.

In all cases the primary responsibility for sorting out student-supervisor problems lies with the university. Problems that cannot be resolved within the panel, the department, or school will inevitably require intervention from the research office or higher. Intervention is never easy, as it involves formal investigation and a decision about where fault, if any, lies. Panel membership can be changed, either through disciplinary or 'no fault' procedures, but should the decision be that the student is at fault, then intervention can mean time out to solve personal problems or acquire specific research training (e.g. research methods). In very serious cases of 'insoluble differences' it can also mean cancellation of the enrolment, subject to appeal mechanisms. Each university will have published regulations about how such cases are handled.

Resources changing

Research projects begin with a research plan that included consideration of the necessary resources, human and financial. What if these are not available, or perhaps more difficult and costly, once they are needed a couple of years later? This is more likely in the part-time research training model we are discussing than with full-time, shorter time-frame projects. This is a problem primarily for the supervisors and the institution, as they signed off on the plan and the resources, although it is also an important part of research training for the student to know how to solve such problems. It is therefore an institutional and supervisor responsibility to advise how to identify and acquire the increased resources, and a research student responsibility to participate in the solution. Supervisors will know of likely funding sources and should direct students to request increases or extensions. As a rule, research projects should not be threatened by this kind of resource issue, as the shortfall is usually small. The exception to this rule is the loss of a genuinely important human resource expertise. Sometimes the loss of a particular source of methodological expertise can be a difficult problem. Again, it is primarily up to the supervisors to use their networks to fill any gaps.

Another kind of resource problem can arise if the research uncovers an interesting, perhaps unexpected, issue that merits further exploration but requires further resources. This situation presents a paradox and a dilemma for researchers. On the one hand this is likely to be a genuinely interesting issue that the student feels has to be answered while he or she is 'on the case'. On the other hand, this may well divert resources and delay the original research plan. The possibility should trigger a full research panel meeting to discuss the advantages and disadvantages of dealing now versus dealing later with this opportunity. In theory, dealing later is the better path for a research student, as that facilitates early completion of the research project and allows for future focus on a project that builds on the original project. That would of course need its own research plan, design and resource acquisition. Just occasionally, the research panel may support dealing now with the opportunity, as it may not require much additional time or resources. If they support doing it now, the supervisors should assist the student to identify and acquire the necessary additional resources and negotiate a new research plan and timeline. Needless to say, family members and work colleagues will need to be consulted and contribute to the decision, as any additional work is likely to impact on them.

Feeling overwhelmed

It is not difficult at times to feel as if 'more has been bitten of than can be chewed'. There are two possible underlying situations. The first is that everything is probably fine, but that the ebb and flow of research, professional work and personal lives simply collide here and there, resulting in a sense that the research is too much to bear. The problem here is predominantly one of project management, and the resolution involves revising project timelines, work schedules, personal and family arrangements, or all of the above.

The second possibility is that the perception is correct and that the research project is too big or too difficult, within the available resources and time-frame. The most likely problem is poor preparation and planning, for which supervisors must share responsibility. Successful research needs, apart from an appropriate research question, methodology, supervision, funding, and a research student with the time, energy and skills to achieve the tasks. One reasonably common challenge is that many potential research students will over-estimate their ability to conduct research and aim for a higher degree than their experience can support. For example, it is common for health professionals, and sometimes their supervisors, to assume that undergraduate research experience is sufficient to start directly into a research masters or even doctoral level research project. In fact this is rarely the case, as few undergraduate degrees include significant depth of research training, but rather some research experience. There are some notable exceptions (e.g. medical graduates who also did an intercalated research year), but most potential research students would benefit from formally studying at least a coursework masters module in qualitative and quantitative research methods.

Even if research students have completed a research methods module, lack of knowledge can still arise, particularly in research projects outside past experience or on the boundary of different research paradigms (e.g. biomedical and education). The resolution lies in recognising this as a problem and doing something about it. Additional help can always be sought, sometimes through the addition of another supervisor with relevant expertise. Books can always be read, and advice can usually be sought from experts in the field. It is essential that any gaps in knowledge and understanding are addressed early, as persisting in some ignorance may well lead to poor outcomes.

The results are different from what was expected

Sound research involves a clear, answerable question or testable hypothesis, the appropriate methods, smooth collection of data or information, smooth analysis and clear outcomes. Well, actually, no, this is not always the case. Research is by definition exploring the unknown, admittedly based on evidence from prior research to guide that exploration. It is therefore prey to the uncertainties that surround life, and a lot of things can happen to interfere with this apparently idyllic process.

Conducting research projects requires a high awareness of how the project is progressing. Projects must be monitored throughout and a keen eye must be kept open to detect early any signs of departure from the expected – that is one of the advantages of the project timeline chart discussed in Chapter 3. Experienced supervisors should be involved in this as they will have seen it happen before. Most of the departures from the expected will have one or more reasons. The analysis may not have worked because the method turned out not to be ideal for the data or information that was collected. The collection of data or information may not have worked because recruitment of participants failed to meet expectations. The research question or testable hypothesis might turn out to be less clear than originally thought, meaning that the research design was not ideal and some vital information was not even sought. A highly relevant piece of information might come to light after the project commenced that, had it been available, might have led to a different research design. Most horrifying of all, someone else might be a year or so ahead of the project, unknown to you, and publish a paper that either answers the question or raises serious questions about the basis of the research. The important issue here for research students is to learn from what happens – after all, this is research training.

While no research student or supervisor wants any of these problems to occur, they will from time to time. It is important to be aware of the possibilities, and to deal with them, because the experience should make the next research project better. The stakes are higher for doctoral level projects, as the time-frame is longer and there are expectations of a reasonably clear and genuinely new outcome. Hence doctoral level research students have additional responsibilities to monitor not only their own projects, but the international literature and the proceedings of research presentations at conferences. A sign of a good doctoral level student is an ability to keep the literature review current and refine research to build on the results of other research that emerge even during the student's own research project.

Occasionally a project will become seriously derailed by either internal (failure to recruit etc.) or external factors, such as a policy change in the health system. One example from the author's experience is a project that explored in part the quality of rural obstetric services. By the time it commenced (a year from funding application) dramatically higher professional indemnity rates caused over 50% of potential rural doctors to cease obstetric services. Rarely a project might have to be abandoned, as experienced researchers can usually adapt research questions and designs, for example to examine the influence of the external policy change. Research students and supervisors may need to work fast and creatively to salvage a reasonable project outcome that meets degree requirements.

On the other hand, not all departures from the expected are negative outcomes. The most interesting results from research projects are often those that do not conform to the expected, as such findings challenge thinking and may lead to genuinely new understandings and concepts. Many of the major research breakthroughs have been almost accidental. One example is the discovery of penicillin mould in some Petri dishes left on a window ledge (by Alexander Fleming), and there are many others.

Falling out of love with the topic

The heading might sound a bit strange, but it probably conveys the message. Success in a research project requires immersion in the topic. As discussed in earlier chapters, the research student pathway is easier if the research topic area is of personal interest. This is more common with experienced health professionals doing applied research that is relevant to their professional practice lives. Research students have to 'live with' their research topics for a considerable time. Students with longer projects, such as those at doctoral level, usually have the most intense 'relationship' with their research topic.

The real test of this interest comes later, when the initial excitement is over and hard work is required. Research students may have to read a huge amount of information about their research topics and become relatively expert in it. Maintaining currency of this expertise requires effort and perhaps a lot of time reading and thinking. Sorting, categorising and analysing data can be assisted by computers, but still require a lot of personal time and thinking. It is quite easy to find some or all of this a bit of a chore, particularly if the research topic is of lesser interest or relevance to other things in life. It is therefore not hard to become bored with the topic and be completely unexcited by the necessary immersion that maintains both currency and the analysis and interpretation of data or information gathered. It is not unheard of for research students to say that they 'hate' their research topic and 'never want' to study that general topic ever again. Loss of interest can still occur when the topic was originally interesting and relevant to professional life, although is less likely.

What can be done if this happens? The best answer probably lies in having a 'vacation' from the research project, switching thinking to other things in life. This is not necessarily easy, as universities may have rules about timelines and completion rates. A break away from research is often easier with longer, doctoral level, projects, as an annual vacation should be factored into every project that is a year or more in length. Even if it is difficult to arrange, a break is much better than ceasing the research project, and students who are seriously disaffected with their project should discuss this with their supervisors.

One or both parties may feel guilty about the failure to maintain what was originally an exciting venture. 'Was it my fault?' is a likely thought. The answer, of course, is that research training should be suspended or even ceased on a 'no fault' basis, as the reasons are usually outside the control of both student and supervisor. In such cases, guilt is unnecessary, although it may require formal counselling for this to be worked through.

Prevention is even better, so choose the research question very carefully! Wherever possible, take plenty of time thinking about the options and choose whatever appeals most. Expect to have fluctuations in interest and build in as much flexibility as time and rules permit.

Becoming obsessed with the topic

The reverse situation is where the topic is so interesting that research students devote too much time to their projects. One feature of research is that it can occupy a lot of 'thinking space', even away from the research project base, and it is not difficult to find oneself thinking about research-related issues during either professional practice time, personal time, or even both. Dinner conversation with family members is difficult if heads are busy thinking about the latest paper or the analysis of data. A balance must be found between too little and too much interest, ideally by trying to clearly separate activities. For example, working at home may be convenient, but can also be intrusive on family life. One way of dealing with this is to work only when young children are in bed asleep, or when partners are busy with their own interests, and other solutions can be found to suit most stages of life. It is likely that a degree of 'obsession' with the research topic is helpful, although the ability to 'switch off' is an essential skill to develop. Research supervisors are not always good role models in this regard, as some successful researchers become very focused on quite narrow research themes and topics. This may be a good thing for senior professional academics, although can result in almost complete absorption into academic life – such people are the inspiration for the clichéd 'nutty' or 'absent minded' professors who seem detached from the rest of the world, pursuing apparently odd interests.

However there are limits to the degree to which research students should allow research training to dominate their lives. The truth is that a research topic is just that – a part of work life – but only a part, and an even smaller part of one's whole life. Achieving this balance can be difficult, but research students who feel that they are becoming too focused on their research should talk with their supervisors or the university student support service.

Writer's block

This is a familiar concept, as it is often claimed by even experienced authors. What it means is that words just do not seem to flow from brain to pen. This can happen at the commencement of writing. But that is probably more related to lack of experience in writing longer documents; this is discussed in Chapter 7. The variety of writer's block discussed here is what experienced authors talk about, where the problem occurs in the middle of a substantial writing task, a most distressing and strange phenomenon.

The cause of this appears to be unknown, and is not related to any genuine neurological or psychological event. What generally happens is that the writer just 'runs out' of things to write. The writer's head is usually full of ideas and concepts, but they whirl around and words do not seem to come out in any logical or flowing manner. In the 'mind's eye' it is possible to see the words, but not the sentences, paragraphs or chapters.

Should this happen, the best solution is probably to have a rest from writing – do something completely different for a while. The time taken to recover is variable, but the writer is aware when recovery is happening, because the thoughts just seem to fall into sentences and suddenly make sense. Taking time out is again more difficult for shorter term projects, but is nevertheless necessary.

Loss of data or drafts of reports

While computers and word processing software are tremendous assets in any writing task, there are traps for the unwary. It is easy to rely on computer memory, but computers can fail due to a range of relatively common events, such as hard drives crashing and computer virus interference. It is not uncommon for drafts of documents to be lost, and this poses a serious challenge, as potentially entire documents have to be re-written.

The solution is simple: have one or more current and accurate back up copies of all documents, whether on another computer, a movable storage device or a server. In particular, keep copies of data or information separate from thesis drafts, so that everything cannot be lost in one incident. Ideally, at least one of these copies should be kept at another location, perhaps in a fireproof safe. This may sound obsessional, but can restore sanity if there is a calamitous loss of everything.

Timelines slipping

It is almost a certainty that a research project will not run exactly as planned. As discussed above, resources might be delayed, personal or family member illness force time out, or work might place additional demands if a colleague cannot contribute an increased share of practice work to cover the absence. Data might come in more slowly or the analysis might be more complex than expected. One or more supervisor might lose interest, be no longer be available, or have a personality clash with the student. The possibilities for delay are considerable, and not always predictable.

Once family, friends and the workplace have accepted that someone valuable will be 'absent' for a defined period of time, any extension of that time because of project delays is likely to be very unpopular. It can also be very frustrating for research students, who mentally allocate a certain amount of time to a project and, towards the end of the allotted time, just want it all over with.

What can be done to prevent delay? Well, some preventative measures are appropriate. Most are about setting honest, realistic, pragmatic and flexible timelines and expectations at home and work, and most importantly, with the research student and the supervisors. It is also wise to have at least one back up plan, and to plan for regular meetings with supervisors so that progress can be carefully monitored and plans can, if necessary, be modified as soon as possible. It may be wise to build in and plan for potential delays and allow time to manage them. If delays do not happen, either a more relaxed pace or an early finish is easier to deal with than the stress of unexpected delays, more hectic work schedules to catch up, or having to extend project timelines. These steps are summarised in Box 6.1.

Box 6.1 Steps to prevent delay in project timelines.

- Make sure you are committed and able to complete the project
- Choose a research question that is interesting and relevant
- Be honest with yourself
- Be honest with family and work colleagues
- Be clear about expectations (style, structure, workload etc.)
- Set realistic timelines
- Build in flexibility and expectation of delay
- Build in vacation periods for longer projects
- Plan generous phase transitions
- Have (several?) pragmatic back up plans

What can be done to minimise the impact of delay? Quite a lot! Think back to the project timeline chart discussed in Chapter 3. This is the key to managing timelines, not just because it forces thinking about timelines, deadlines and sequencing of research phases, but because timeline slippage should be built in to the project timeline. It is wise to plan for 'transition periods' where phases overlap. For example, allow generous time for the literature review and project design phase, so that the data collection can start on time. Be clear about what is expected in terms of writing and referencing style, size and structure of the thesis, as changing those retrospectively can be very time consuming. Ideally, plan a short break before data collection starts. It may not eventuate, but it does allow for timeline slippage. Plan for the write up phase to commence after data analysis, but aim to have the first half of the thesis (background, literature review and methods) written before that point. Monitor progress regularly – having the project plan as a highly visible chart on the wall is a good idea – and report any likely deviation early. Report problems with supervisors to the person in the institution with the 'research monitor' role. Be honest and keep family and work informed. Be prepared to switch to a back up plan if the original timeline becomes impossible. These steps are summarised in Box 6.2.

Box 6.2 Steps to minimise impact of delay in project timelines.

- Check progress against the plan regularly
- Seek early advice from supervisors if delay looms
- Get ahead with writing the first half of the thesis
- If supervisor relationships are poor, seek advice from the 'research monitor'
- Keep family and work colleagues informed
- Modify research plans as soon as the need becomes clear

Case studies

Our three research students have been working hard on their respective projects which, although all quite different from each other, pose similar kinds of challenges. Jamie has always had the most complex personal circumstances, and perhaps the most complex topic, so it is not surprising that he will encounter some problems refining his ideas amidst a busy work and home life. Ahmed has fewer family complexities, but has chosen a brave research topic that spans professions and methodologies. While this can be fascinating and can result in interesting and worthwhile results, not all academics and professionals will see the point. Susan has always been the most experienced and capable researcher, with the clearer research topic, and she is in much greater control of her research project. Thankfully, her supervisors recognise and facilitate this.

Case A

Jamie's project is proceeding amidst some turmoil at work and at home. He is married with three young children, all at primary school, and is used to doing a share of the home duties. He is finding it very difficult to balance his life, and all participants seem to feel that they are getting the raw end of the deal. His work colleagues are supportive, but mutter at meetings that Jamie is not really doing his fair share. He is successful in gaining a small research grant from the GP training School, and is allowed to spend some of his funded training time on the research project, but the practice has had difficulty finding a stable locum arrangement to replace his sessions, as the research demands require some flexibility. His application to other funding sources fails, mainly because the priorities were in clinical, rather than education, research. The family is supportive, but he is actually working more hours each week than he thought and they feel he is not there for them when needed. He finds that he has to do quite a bit of reading and thinking at home, and this sometimes gets in the way of activities with his children and sleep. His partner is also a busy career person, and feels that the pressure on her is just too much. Jamie becomes quite stressed out and feels that he should give up research training and return to his former, more acceptably balanced life. His supervisors detect this pressure (it is generally obvious!) and arrange a series of meetings where they discuss the options. The mutually agreed decision (agreed also by work and home!) is that Jamie will take three months off to relieve the pressure and allow renegotiation of commitments at home and work. He can then resume, hopefully better prepared to commit time in a more balanced way.

Jamie's work and family circumstances become more manageable and he returns to the project with more family support and a lesser practice contribution. It is never easy, but he manages to find a reasonable middle path that allows for a manageable balance between practice, research and home activity. The project goes well and Jamie is able to collect information that improves understanding of why some learners respond so differently to feedback. For some there appears to be a connection between negative response to feedback and lack of insight into personal performance. The project takes him a little into cognitive psychology, a discipline that is quite new to him. He recognises this and seeks advice, eventually linking with an academic psychologist in the university. He presents his findings at a medical education conference, and is encouraged to write a paper for a national medical education journal. His work is publicised by his college as 'groundbreaking' and attracts the attention of the chair of the professional regulatory authority, which is seeking ways of better measuring poor professional performance.

Case B

After three months Ahmed is troubled because he feels he is not really 'connecting' with his supervisors. He is having no trouble finding the time for his research, as he has a supportive partner and no children, and his employer has released him on paid leave for one day each week to focus on the research. He feels that he has a reasonable relationship with each of his supervisors, but the nursing academic appears to be not at all interested in the management flow methodology issues in the research, but totally fixed on clinical nursing aspects. The management academic is the reverse of this – no interest in clinical nursing and a narrow interest in complex decision theory that does not often seem relevant to professional practice. The two do not get on well and Ahmed is having great difficulty getting them to agree or to even meet together with him. The nursing academic (the primary supervisor) advises Ahmed that the project is starting to look nothing like a nursing research project and that unless Ahmed changes back to clearer nursing research he will withdraw from the supervision panel. Further, a comment is made that promotion within nursing will be very difficult if he continues on this odd tangential path. Ahmed finds this stressful as he thinks he can still see where nursing meets management research, and he knows that his supervisor is often on promotion panels. His partner is a good listener who suggests that he goes to the research monitor for advice. The research monitor speaks with both supervisors and finds that they never really agreed on how to mix professions and methodologies. The research monitor agrees that the project is viable if the student is willing to persist, and recommends another supervisor, a nursing academic who is relatively new to the department but quite open to the underlying concepts of the research. The more senior nursing academic agrees to reduce involvement and focus on generic research issues rather than the content. The medical director also agrees to be a little more involved, although mostly for clinical advice, as she has little direct research experience. This appears to be a satisfactory arrangement. Over the next few months Ahmed works well with his new supervision panel and feels he has gained from having supervisors with such different expertise. He believes that he has been able to maintain the nursing professional relevance and insert some management expertise to develop a system that monitors and manages patient flows in a triage system. He and his supervisors are confident of a sound outcome.

Case C

Susan is powering ahead and doing well. She was successful in her application for two days each week free of normal professional duties, one paid for by her employer and the other funded as a part-time research fellowship through the College of Speech and Language Therapists. She has a supportive partner and her children are at secondary school, allowing her to devote the two full days a week to her research. However, about 12 months into the project her father is found to have rectal cancer. She decides to take a few weeks off to deal with that, and the supervisors agree as she is ahead of her project plan. The surgery goes well and the prognosis turns out to be better than feared, and Susan's family advise her to continue with the research. However she is aware that he could worsen at any time and discusses with her family how they might manage any recurrence. As part of this, her employer agrees her time commitment could be reduced if necessary. While she was more involved with her father's illness, Susan still occasionally read the literature and she found a fascinating new paper that was very relevant to her project, so she emailed the international authors and obtained permission to include aspects of their work as comparison in her project. Her supervisors were happy with this as it would make the project more current without adding complexity or cost. Susan's father became terminally ill and died about a year later. She took some time off again, but with the planned additional support managed to stay reasonably on track.

Conclusion

Research, not to mention life in general, is subject to all the dynamics that facilitate or impede progress along a planned pathway. It is almost inevitable that research projects and research training will encounter difficulties, of which there are many kinds. The best approach is to predict problems, try to prevent them, and to intervene early if any arise, using the support of the research supervision panel, family, friends and the workplace. With careful planning and use of the available support resources, the potential 'roller coaster ride' should have fewer steep rises and falls. For some, encountering and solving problems is all part of the excitement of research.

Chapter 7

Assessment of research performance

The success of discovery depends upon the time of its appearance.

S Weir Mitchell 1928

Introduction

Many issues that can arise during research supervision are highly dependent on the nature of the particular research project. Research projects are so varied that issues relating to the detail of each project, such as methodological and interpretation issues, will have to be resolved by discussion with the supervisors. This book cannot deal in detail with all of the possible issues that will arise, because they are so context specific. We therefore now turn to the final major stage of research training – formal assessment of the research candidature.

Assessment of research training achievement is in principle similar to the assessment of any training programme: there is formative assessment, summative assessment, and in-training assessment. The assessment methods should match the learning objectives and tasks of research training, and may reflect the assessment of components of research, which could be regarded as research competencies. These include accessing, understanding and synthesising the literature, framing a researchable question or testable hypothesis, selecting the most appropriate methods in designing a project, analysing and interpreting data or information, and reporting of results.

These research competencies are usually measured by a combination of within training and end of training assessment. Within training assessment may include the original research proposal, drafts of literature reviews, confirmation and exit seminars, a written product (thesis or portfolio) and some form of oral defence of a presentation of the research project. All of these involve varying degrees of peer review, both internal and external. Recently the emphasis has moved from reliance on a major endpoint assessment (e.g. a large thesis) to multiple, smaller assessments both during and at the end of the research training candidature. This is a much better approach, as research students receive more feedback on how they are progressing and are much less likely to submit a failing thesis. This chapter discusses the assessment methods commonly used for research candidature and offers advice on how to approach them.

Within training assessment

There are several potential within training assessments, not all of which are used all of the time by all universities. Some have been discussed briefly in earlier chapters. Some may be used for purely 'formative' assessment, meaning that their main role is to guide the development of students through provision of constructive feedback. A variant of this is that an activity may be a 'hurdle': that is, something that must be done before proceeding to the next step, but does not contribute directly to a final decision on meeting degree requirements. Others may be 'summative' assessment: that is an assessment that can be used for feedback purposes, but is scored formally and required to be included with the endpoint assessment products. The range of possibilities is listed in Box 7.1.

Box 7.1 Within training assessable research products.

Initial research project proposal
Early draft of the literature
Research grant application
Ethics application
Confirmation and/or exit seminars

The initial research proposal and an early draft of a literature review are usually both formative assessment and hurdles that determine eligibility to proceed. The standards expected here are not necessarily high, although they are for higher level degrees, and supervisors usually provide detailed feedback that aims to improve the students' awareness of the research topic and how to access relevant literature and form appropriate research questions.

A research grant application, when it is necessary, may be a requirement for conducting the research, but is generally not formally assessed. This may be a missed opportunity, because research grantsmanship is a difficult set of skills that may be best developed through early and regular experience and formal assessment. It is often assumed that research graduates have strong research grant writing skills, but this is often not the case. Ethics applications are another absolute hurdle, without which research projects cannot proceed, but are also often not formally assessed. Again, this is a research skill that may well benefit from nurturing and more formal assessment.

The most commonly included formal assessment during research training is assessment of academic presentation skills. In the traditional 'big thesis' model of research training assessment, the assessment of a presentation at the beginning or the end of the research (or both) is usually a formative hurdle. However, in the more modern portfolio approach to research training assessment, inclusion of a peer reviewed conference presentation is often encouraged or even required (see below). Oral and poster presentation skills are quite different from those required to produce a written research product, and may require some development.

Oral presentation skills

Oral presentations are one of the most commonly used activities by academics, and yet also one of the least taught; this is the strongest argument in favour of making oral presentations part of research training assessment. A research presentation is much more than an expert providing new information. In addition, oral presentations require this information to be provided in a relevant, meaningful and memorable way.

Some tips are listed in Box 7.2, falling into several categories. The first category is about being prepared, through planning the session carefully, getting timings right, and pacing the stages of the presentation. The second category is about knowing the project and the literature well, sounding like you know it well and being able to pitch the contents at the level of all present, from novice to experts. The third category is about the technicalities of the presentation software: numbers of slides, uncrowded and meaningful slides, appropriate use of images and diagrams and avoidance of too many audio-visual tricks. The final category is about presenter behaviour – animated, interested, dynamic, mobile, attentive to the audience and wanting to improve mutual understanding through interaction. The question time is very important, because this combines all three categories, and it is where assessors will judge ability to understand the topic in depth and to respond at the appropriate level to searching questions.

Box 7.2 Oral presentation skills for a one-hour seminar.

- Plan the session very carefully and perform it in practice with peers
- Ensure that you finish in no later than 40 minutes to leave time for questions and discussion
- Never run over time
- Know the relevant literature very well: speak from a position of authority
- The audience may include experts to novices: adjust messages to all levels
- Use no more than 25–30 slides during a 50 minute session
- Use font size 24 at a minimum on slides
- Have no more than 4 bullet points on a presentation slide
- If relevant, use a limited number of clinical healthcare images to raise interest
- Use diagrams and figures to summarise complex conceptual issues
- Avoid using too many fancy features (too many colours, sounds, video etc.) as this may detract from the underlying message
- Never use a slide that is over-crowded and say 'you probably can't read this as it is too busy'. Design slides that are meaningful
- Never just read the slides: your oral presentation should elaborate the information on them
- Be animated, move around, ask questions and maintain eye contact with the audience
- Avoid turning lights down too far so that you can maintain eye contact with the audience
- Carefully observe audience behaviour; adjust your presentation if they look bored or sleepy
- Provide presentation handouts and encourage the audience to provide feedback

It is very wise to practice a presentation, ideally with a friendly audience of fellow practitioners and researchers, and repeat this until you feel comfortable. Try to adjust to being the object of attention of an audience sitting in a darkened room, where you may have difficulty picking up body language. Expect some difficult questions from a variety of areas of the presentation, and ask your friendly audience to ask you really difficult questions. In fact, think of the questions you would not like to be asked, and arrange for someone to ask that in the practice sessions. It is likely that someone will ask it in the real presentation.

Poster presentation skills

Conference poster sessions are an important way of communicating a lot of information from several brief presentations. Formats vary, but generally involve themed sessions where researchers present their work to an audience of like-minded fellow researchers. In some formats each presenter may be allowed to speak briefly, either in front of their poster or at a brief plenary where all presenters speak briefly and show perhaps one or two slides. Posters are ideal for reporting research ideas and concepts, planned or half-completed projects, or the results of small projects.

Designing a conference poster is however not as easy as it sounds. There is an absolute limit on space for words, images and diagrams, and yet the poster may have to include all Introduction, Methods, Results and Discussion (IMRAD) headings plus some key references. There are two general approaches – design your own or pay for a designer and formatter who takes your information electronically and sends back a colour printed poster. The latter is easier and often a better product, but is much more expensive, unless the research organisation has access to in-house resources, such as the appropriate software and an A2 colour printer and laminator.

Some tips for the DIY approach are similar to those for oral presentations. Plan the poster carefully and include in this planning a practice presentation. Consider the distance away that readers will stand and design sections of the

---

Box 7.3 Oral presentation skills for a one-hour seminar.

- Plan the poster carefully, and aim to include a 'whole' story within available space
- Use plain language that tells the story simply
- Use font sizes that can be read from about 1.5 metres distance
- Demonstrate mastery of the literature and issues
- Pitch messages at the most likely audience – fellow researchers?
- If relevant, use perhaps one relevant clinical healthcare image to raise interest
- Use perhaps one or two diagrams and figures to summarise complex conceptual issues
- Avoid clashing or too many colours
- Provide handouts and an email address and encourage debate with the audience

poster accordingly, with appropriate font size etc. Use images and diagrams sparingly, when they say things more easily or in less space than words can achieve. Be careful of colours so that meaning is enhanced, not distracted from. The tips are summarised in Box 7.3.

End of training assessment

No research project is complete without some form of reporting on what happened and what was found, because all researchers rely on research reports to plan further research to extend knowledge and understanding. In research training, degrees will not be awarded without some form of reporting, and the higher the level of the degree, the higher are the reporting expectations.

Theses and portfolios

The first kind of report is a monograph that describes the whole research project in some detail. This is generally the thesis that is submitted for measurement of successful research candidature, and is therefore mandatory. The institution will have guidelines for word limits, reference style and formatting that have to be followed. The traditional approach is a single body of work in IMRAD format with expected lengths measured in the number of words. The size and weight of the thesis depends on the level of the degree (larger for doctoral level theses) and the field of research (longer in the humanities). In the health professions a bachelor honours thesis might be as few as 10–20 000 words, a masters level thesis around 30–60 000 words, and a doctoral level thesis around 60–100 000 words, but there are wide variations, and the rules of the particular university must be adhered to.

Increasingly, theses may be allowed to diverge from the traditional model and include multiple products that might reflect the precise nature of the project. A major weakness of formal theses is that only a few copies are ever printed – one in the university library, a copy for each supervisor and a few for the research graduates' bookshelves. Hence their contents are inaccessible to people outside a very small network. In response, universities are adopting a variety of more accessible research products as part of the formal assessment of research achievement, as listed in Box 7.4.

One approach is to encourage submission of papers published externally in academic journals prior to awarding the degree. The research student then

---

Box 7.4 End of training assessable research products.

Traditional large, single concept thesis
A small book compilation of published papers or expanded versions as chapters
Portfolio of different, discrete components reflecting mutiple research tasks
Inclusion of different formats and electronic media, such as CD-ROMs, DVDs etc.

compiles and submits either copies of the published paper with some form of relatively brief narrative that explains the context and linkages between the papers, or an expanded version of each published paper in a small monograph. This is sometimes published formally as a small book, with an ISBN number so that it can be traced and purchased.

Another approach is to require a thesis to include several smaller, defined research products, such as a literature review, a peer reviewed conference paper presentation, a peer reviewed journal paper, a chapter of book, or interactive audio-visual material on CD-ROMs and DVDs. These discrete research products may be all about a single research project, but increasingly are allowed to reflect more than one research project, which is ideal for professional doctorates. This form of thesis is often called a research portfolio. While some traditional academics resist the move away from the traditional big thesis, there are clear advantages in the more recent developments in the way in which research outcomes are communicated more effectively and more widely.

Getting started on the thesis

Writing can be the hardest part of being a research student. Most health professionals have achieved well in science-based subjects, which are not known for requiring reading long books or writing long essays of flowing prose. Indeed, the opposite is generally true: scientific writing is concise and highly structured. Higher word limits and more detailed discussion is often more appropriate in medical humanities and education projects, which tend to use qualitative methods, as the rules depend on the broad research paradigm more than the specific topic. At the beginning of a research training project many students may be well out of practice at writing anything more than brief, concise (almost terse) paragraphs in patient records, referral letters, or patient reports. Recently the writing of letters and reports has often been aided by 'filling in' document frameworks that automatically extract much of the relevant information from computerised patient record systems. The requirement to write some form of coherent thesis, whether 10 000 or 60 000 words in length, can be terrifying!

The best way to work on documents is to have a draft to work from, and guess where this draft has to come from? The answer is the research student him or herself. The good news is that the first draft can be just a whole lot of words thrown together, with loose headings and dot points. No one else need see this, and there is no embarrassment in having poorly connected, loose ideas that are written in ungrammatical language. It almost does not matter that this first draft may be a jumble of words that may need to be moved to other headings. Word processors are fantastic tools as wording can be cut and pasted wherever needed as the document is refined.

One simple method that some beginners find helpful is to start by writing a list of probable chapter and section headings. The IMRAD format provides probable chapter headings, although most thesis formats will also require chapter numbers, such as Chapter 1: Introduction etc. Under each chapter heading, consider the most likely sub-headings and just jot them down as a rough guide. It may be possible to generate an indicative table of contents, which can then be expanded, point by point, but in any sequence. How to structure a thesis is discussed further below.

Something that is not often appreciated by novice writers of even scientific literature is that writing is essentially a creative task. It is very hard to sit at a desk and tap away at a computer unless one is 'in the mood'. Most novice writers will tell tales of trying to do this, often because of looming deadlines, and finding that the words just do not seem to flow. This is sometimes confused with 'writer's block' (see Chapter 6), but is actually different from a barrier to writing that successful writers encounter in the middle of a manuscript. In this situation it is more about inexperience leading to a novice writer not understanding what it takes to write a substantial document.

Box 7.5 Tips for writing.

- Warn family, friends and colleagues that you are in writing mode
- Use a quiet, distraction free room to write
- Allocate protected time to think and write
- Use other activities to think about what you need to write
- Formulate wording in your head
- Write when you feel as if the words are ready to come out
- Be prepared to write down what comes out, and revise this later
- Keep multiple back up copies of what you write

The ability to write may be related to personality types and learning styles, and there is almost certainly no single approach that works for everybody. Some tips for 'getting in the mood' are presented in Box 7.5. Writing is not a disconnected task – it is the result of thinking through what has to be said. The most important part of writing is thinking through the research project, sifting information and formulating sentences and paragraphs in your mind. When these words seem to make sense, go to a computer and type them, in any order or sequence, attached to whatever sub-heading seems the most relevant. Things can be shifted around later.

The coming together of ideas into words is unpredictable. You may have to be prepared to write at odd times. For example, it is possible to wake up early with an apparently wonderful set of words in your mind, which are best captured immediately: later you may not remember them. Writing can be an intense and apparently lonely phase, and it is wise to warn loved ones that you might suddenly disappear and tap away for a while. Once a writer is 'in the mood', writing speeds up and the quality of first drafts improves, so once you are 'in the mood', try to stay there for a while. Finally, have multiple back ups of what you write, as it is extremely frustrating to have to re-write sections and quite likely that the original version was the most inspired. There are simple ways of doing this, such as turning on the automatic save function to every 10–15 minutes (minimising potential loss) and ALWAYS copying drafts to another storage device.

Structuring a thesis

Theses often have the traditional IMRAD format, although the requirements of each university will make formatting issues clear. The introduction is a very important part of a thesis, because it tells readers why the research was done, where the ideas or motivation came from and the relevance to the world outside, in this case often to the health care system and perhaps patient care. It is usual to start with an explanation of the general research topic area, why this is of interest and relevance, why this has (if it has!) attracted personal interest, a summary of the general context of the research topic (e.g. potential impact on health care), a summary of the broad research question(s), and an outline of the rest of the thesis. A formal literature review is part of the introduction, but is likely to require its own separate chapter (Chapter 2: Literature Review). The literature is then summarised under sub-headings that make sense to the researcher (and is likely to make sense to the readers), and that will depend on the topic. Use of any new research methods (or different use of existing methods) will also need discussion and referencing to the academic literature. Sometimes the literature review is so large or complex that it requires two chapters.

The method chapter (Chapter 3 or 4) almost writes itself. This chapter should begin with the specific research question(s) or testable hypotheses, explain the methods chosen, and then contain a simple description of the research design. The latter is usually made easier by the inclusion of flow diagrams and figures that display the phases in sequence. Some justification of the methods chosen is required if this has not been dealt with in the literature review.

Research students should be encouraged to write drafts of these first three to four chapters quite early, perhaps even before data or information is collected, as this gets a lot of work out of the way at a time when the contents of these chapters is freshest in their minds. Words, paragraphs, and whole sub-sections can be moved around later.

The next chapter is usually a presentation of the results, followed by a chapter which discusses the results. Here there is some room for variation, again depending on the nature of the research. Sometimes this extreme separation of results (factual details) and discussion (interpretation and meaning) is required, particularly for more pure science research. On the other hand, it often makes sense to combine the factual details with the interpretation and meaning, an approach which leads to two or more separate chapters that may be themed according to a logical grouping of the results. For example, if a research project has two or three connected sections or stages, perhaps using different methods, then these can be presented separately with results and discussion combined. Supervisors are the best source of advice about which method is best suited to the particular project and the research field.

Arguably the most important chapter is that which explores the meaning of the research outcome and links it back to the literature and the original research question(s). This is called the 'so what' factor in research – the implications for the research community, the health care system and perhaps patient care. It is important to acknowledge the limitations of the research, as research projects generally cannot deal with all possible contexts and variables, and reviewers will expect to see that research students understand what can and cannot be achieved through research. It is also important to generate some ideas about future research questions that will build on this particular project and lead to further enhancement of knowledge and understanding. The most informed research questions generally come from those with a strong understanding of how current knowledge and understanding was achieved. Some reviewers say that the most important chapters are the first and last, as they are what link research to the real world.

Avoiding plagiarism

Plagiarism is currently a hot topic, and yet is poorly understood. Plagiarism really means that information is included in any information source without appropriate referencing. This means that the word covers a spectrum of problems from deliberate cheating through to poor referencing skills.

All research students should become very familiar with the plagiarism definitions, policies and rules of their university, because the penalties for transgression can be severe, up to and including expulsion from the degree programme with no credit. Such penalties are reserved for larger scale, deliberate cheating, judged through complex processes that are subject to appeal. Cause for the more severe penalties would include falsifying results or using long passages of wording from the papers or theses of other researchers as if the words were those of the writer. Both are clearly wrong and deserve serious penalty. A more recent variant is where a student pays someone to write their thesis for them and then submits it as personal effort. This is also clearly wrong, but sadly appears not to be infrequent, as websites openly advertise such services for a relatively modest fee. Some students who struggle to write in a second or third language have been tempted to seek such 'assistance' to overcome an understandable problem. The more obvious cheating is often easily detected, as reviewers are familiar with the work being cited (or not) and there are stories of reviewers recognising their own wording in theses they are asked to mark.

There are simple ways of avoiding lesser transgressions. There are rules about how to use the wording of others (word limits, indenting, using italics etc.). Most universities also make available plagiarism software, such as TURNITIN (www.turnitin.com), which scans documents and provides feedback on percentage of words matching the literature bank and referencing format. Such software is best used formatively, providing feedback to students on the quality of their writing, so that problems can be addressed before final submission. The percentage of matching words is itself not necessarily important, as research in narrower topics will probably use similar wording to other research products, but it is still a guide to the originality of the writing.

Editing and proofreading

It is worth saying more about these two often forgotten issues. Not so long ago researchers would pay for typists to translate their handwritten notes into reports and papers, but more recently they are more likely to use word processors themselves. Indeed academics have had to become multi-skilled! This is however risky, as most academics are not skilled touch typists and have not been to secretarial college. As a group, academics may be pedantic about the outcomes (more on that later), but they may not have the skills to personally produce a perfect thesis that is grammatically correct and properly formatted. Failure to present a thesis properly is a bit like trying to sell a dirty car with dents in the panels, and will almost certainly cause thesis scorers to make totally avoidable adverse comments.

As a result the revision of draft documents is, as much as anything, an exercise in editing. Ideally, this editing is based on feedback from others who read the manuscript carefully and make detailed notes of typographical errors or potentially ambiguous, unclear or confusing wording. This is essential to the development of a quality product, a judgment that will be made partially on grammar, spelling and formatting, as well as the intrinsic academic merit of the project. It is generally true that writers cannot proofread their own work, because they know what it is supposed to say and may not recognise problems.

There are two kinds of proofreaders, and both should be used. The first is the 'macro' proofreader, who focuses on the project itself, standing back from wording and grammar issues and understanding why the project was done, where it began, how well it is linked to the literature, how well data or information was analysed and interpreted, and how well results were linked back to the literature. This is usually another academic with an understanding of the research topic, although any experienced researcher can provide generic advice and quite often an 'outsider' to the research topic can be more helpful, as any thesis or paper should make sense to a more general audience. Macro proofreaders generally do not even notice typos or spelling mistakes, as their minds sort of 'fill in' small gaps in larger pictures. Their comments will be about 'making sense' overall.

The second kind of proofreader is a person who can spot the smaller typos, spelling mistakes, the use of semi-colons etc. Word processors contain spelling and grammar checking tools, and these should be used, but they miss many small errors, such as words with correct spelling but in the wrong place. It is therefore important to use a proofreader who will notice these problems. Such people will often not be academics (few academics have this skill) and will not necessarily understand the report, but they will ensure that the final product is correctly formatted and has no simple spelling or grammatical errors, avoiding the really embarrassing situation where reviewers provide feedback such as 'full of typos and unfit in its current form'.

Version control

One potential disadvantage of storing multiple copies of draft documents is that it is easy to start further work on an older version of the document. This is not a catastrophic event, but can be difficult to repair if not recognised early. The result can be a hotchpotch document that includes a difficult-to-track combination of final, better draft material and early, incomplete draft material. It is wise to carefully name documents, store them carefully and to choose carefully the latest version of the document for further work.

The thesis review process

Research degrees are awarded on the basis of judgments made by reviewers, in much the same way as editors make decisions about whether or not to publish books or academic papers. The precise details of the process may vary between universities, and research students should ensure that they understand the requirements and assessment process at their particular university, but here is a summary of the generic approach that most universities will adopt, with some variations.

The thesis is not submitted for review until the supervisors believe that it is ready for external scrutiny. The process of internal review and revision can be time consuming but is important, as it is preferable to detect and fix any errors or ambiguities before submission.

A short time (perhaps three months) before the due date for submission, the research student office will contact the supervisors to ascertain the likely date of submission of the thesis. At this time the supervisors will also be asked to nominate a panel of potential reviewers of the thesis. In most cases the research student does not have any formal say in this choice, but in practice most supervisors will discuss the options. This is an important step because the reviewers should not have any prior involvement in the research project, so if the student involved any researchers external to the supervision panel in their project (discussion of research questions, design or interpretation), they should not be nominated. This can be quite constraining with doctoral level degrees in narrow specialised areas, as the international pool of experts may be relatively small. The number of nominated potential reviewers should be at least three more than needed, because some will be unavailable.

Different universities and different level research degrees have different rules about numbers and source of reviewers. As a rule, bachelor (honours) projects might go to a single reviewer, who may be a member of staff at the host university or another university. Masters level degrees generally require two reviewers, one of whom must be external to the host university. PhD theses generally go to two or three reviewers, of whom one may be from the host university and the others external; all must be recognised experts in the relevant field of research. Higher doctorates generally require all reviewers to be external, often international, and all must be recognised experts in the relevant field of research.

The research student office will contact the nominated potential reviewers and make the final choice of the panel membership based on availability to complete the task within a defined period of time, often 6–8 weeks. Time-frames are deliberately short as it is in everybody's interests to have theses dealt with in a timely manner. Some universities offer a modest fee to reviewers for their time, others do not, but either way it is something that academics do for little or no direct reward, but rather as a contribution to the enhancement of knowledge within their field of interest. Most are very happy to do this, as they know that others have to read theses of their own students. Although those with common research interests are often well networked, supervisors do not directly contact the reviewers about theses: this is another important step that avoids any semblance of pressure being placed on reviewers through 'old boy' networks. The final list of reviewers is decided by the research student office.

When the thesis is complete and both student and supervisor are happy with it, it is temporarily bound, with a copy for each reviewer plus a couple of spares. The research student office sends one copy to each of the confirmed reviewers, along with a copy of the degree requirements and how the thesis should be judged. They are asked to read the thesis and complete a form ticking a box adjacent to one of either three or four statements, worded similarly to those listed in Box 7.6. They are also invited to provide detailed comments on any suggestions for amendment or correction.

Clearly all students and supervisors aim for receiving a tick against the first statement – a clear pass. However this is unusual, because by nature most

---

Box 7.6 Thesis reviewer scoring.

- The thesis meets all requirements for the degree, needs no revision or correction, and the degree should be awarded.
- The thesis meets all requirements for the degree, but would benefit from a few minor corrections or voluntary amendments for the student to consider in discussion with supervisors, and with no need to have further external review.
- The thesis meets most requirements, but has some correctable faults that must be addressed before being reviewed externally again.
- The thesis fails to meet the requirements for the degree and has so many faults that it should be completely revised and re-submitted at some future date.

---

academics are pedantic and can find something to suggest. This is where having very good proofreaders is helpful, as having several minor typographical or spelling errors can really upset some reviewers!

In reality, the best grade to hope for is the second – pass with consideration of minor changes without further external review. This is usually left up to the supervisory panel to oversee, and this is usually relatively painless. Most of the suggested corrections will be recommended rather than mandatory, in discussion with supervisors.

The third grade is a disappointment, but is usually able to be resolved satisfactorily. The main problem is that this takes a lot of work and more time, as the corrections have to be made, the thesis re-bound temporarily, and then sent off for external review to at least one of the original external reviewers. The time for this to happen is usually at least three to six months.

The fourth grade is generally taken as a cruel blow, as it really means up to another year of reviewing the data or information, revision in light of the criticism and re-submission. The same reviewers read the re-submission, and they will often expect adherence to their comments and suggestions. This is an unusual and preventable outcome.

Some universities include an additional grade, with words to the effect that the thesis is so poor that it is not salvageable and not even worth revision and re-submission. This is a rare, but obviously disastrous outcome. Again, it should be preventable.

Where the grade is the fourth, and the re-submission is still given a poor grade, or where the recommendation is an outright fail (the fifth grade that is sometimes allowed), the student and supervisors have only one recourse after due consideration of the comments and revision – an appeal that requests either an additional external examiner or an oral defence of the thesis (more of the latter below). To achieve this the case will have to be made that the grades are too harsh through misunderstanding or bias.

Responding to reviewer feedback

Reviewer feedback to all forms of academic publishing, whether for journal papers, books or theses, can come in many varieties. There can be a wide spectrum from effusive positive comments, to neutral and to bitterly critical comments. Some can be rather vague, in fact so vague as to be difficult to interpret, while others can be pedantically precise to the point of aggravation. The comments might come from people who have an open mind and enjoy reading contributions to an international debate, while others might have strong beliefs and do not like reading the work of upstarts who might venture discussion that disagrees with their views. Academics are a very varied group of people, and their feedback can reflect this variety.

However, the point to remember here is that the reviewers were chosen because of their content and/or process expertise and their willingness to do the job. Therefore, the comments of all reviewers need to be taken seriously, carefully considered, and responded to in due course, even if they are advisory rather than mandatory. Peer review is a cornerstone of academic standards, and it is usually well intentioned and reasonably accurate, no matter how upsetting it might be to research students who just want to get past this step and get on with their lives. The substance of the criticism is almost always worth considering, and the result after revision is almost always an improvement.

Sometimes the comments can be in rather harsh wording and be potentially offensive. This is an unfortunate part of the make up of many academics – pedantic, concise to the point of terseness or rudeness, but often correct, at least in part. Part of research training is to learn to accept such criticisms for what they are intended to be. If the comments are upsetting, part (much?) of the reason is really that the end is so close and yet another frustrating hurdle is placed in the way. If there is a lot of work required in considering and responding to the comments, then it may well be advisable to take some time out to think of other things before tackling the task and getting it done. Coming back with a fresh mind can make this both more enjoyable and more achievable.

It is a formal requirement of peer review processes, whether for journals, books or theses, that all comments of all reviewers are listed with a response. For less serious comments, the response might be something like: 'I have discussed this issue with my supervisors and on reflection we think that the original wording is acceptable'. Such a response (disagreeing politely with the reviewer) may be acceptable. In other cases, the response should indicate precisely how wording was changed to reflect different interpretation or discussion of findings, or to include additional references.

In rare circumstances one of the reviewers may provide critical comments that indicate that they completely misunderstood the thesis or have a personal bias that is beyond the usual academic pedantry, perhaps through challenging their own research. Potential reviewers should not accept invitations to review theses where they recognise potential conflict of interest through bias, but some might. This is a very difficult situation to deal with, and will require strong intervention by supervisory panel members to have either an additional reviewer invited to arbitrate (more common) or the particular reviewer over-ruled (uncommon).

Oral defence of a thesis

Some universities also require a public meeting with supervisors and external assessors, at which the thesis is presented by the research student and questions are asked to test the student's understanding. This is more common with doctoral level theses, and is more likely in certain countries (e.g. Europe) than others. In some universities it is a more major determinant of the outcome than the thesis itself, in others it is simply an option when there is serious disagreement amongst thesis reviewers, as mentioned above.

While some might find the thought of an oral defence more appealing than writing a big thesis, it is by no means an easy ride. The defence can take half a day and the assessors can ask very searching questions that have to be answered without being able to access other resources. Many health professionals will have been through viva voce examinations, and an oral defence is a very long and searching version of that process. For many, the stress can be very high. On the other hand, for those research students who have done their work well and know their thesis well, the oral defence can be relatively straightforward.

Reporting to funders and stakeholders

There are other kinds of reports that, while not part of the academic assessment of research training, are required to meet responsibilities to the broader community. These are, as listed in Table 7.1: a report to participants in the research (if any); a report to external stakeholders in the research; a report to the funders of the project; and a report to the ethics committee. The first two are currently optional, although may well become mandatory, but in any case reflect good research practice. The latter two are usually mandatory, and universities may not award degrees until they have been submitted and approved by their relevant organisations.

Table 7.1 Reports not directly contributing to research assessment.

Report	Mandatory
Report to participants in the research	No
Report to stakeholder organisations	No
Report to funders of the research	Yes
Report to the ethics committee	Yes

The report to participants is a nice gesture that is well received by those who provided data or information and, in many ways, allowed the research to happen, often through considerable personal effort that was not financially rewarded. This form of report is usually a very brief (two to three page) summary, de-identified, explaining the main findings that came from the contribution of the participants. Should academic papers result from the research, it is also appropriate to let these people know and perhaps even send them a copy. Participants like to see what came of their contributions and feel appreciated when they see this.

The report to stakeholders is more formal, and could take the form of an executive summary of the thesis. The main objective is to satisfy stakeholders (e.g. hospitals, health authorities, professional bodies or patient groups) that the research project was conducted as intended and completed. Again, notice of any papers or conference presentations can help indicate the impact of the research. These reports are likely to be formally received by stakeholders and may be disseminated through their networks. Again, they are usually well received and make organisations feel as if their support was appreciated.

The report to the research funders of a research project is a mandatory requirement. It focuses on resource use and outcomes – a kind of cost-impact-efficiency report – and has two parts. The first is an audited statement that demonstrates appropriate acquittal of the research grant. This statement comes from the central university administration, although is usually checked by an external auditor. Prudent management of research grants should prevent any difficulties obtaining this document. The second part is a summary of the research project, and this can be the same as that sent to stakeholders: this reduces the potential workload by having only one substantial summarised report of the project. Some funders will also follow up research grant holders several months later to find out what impact the research they funded has had on the broader academic community, in the form of conference presentations, academic papers, books etc.

The final report is to the ethics committee that gave initial approval to commence the research project. This report is often a form to complete, indicating formally that the project was completed and that no ethical issues arose. On the other hand, where ethical issues did arise, a description will be required of the issues and how they were managed.

Case studies

Our three research students have submitted their theses and await decisions by their universities.

Case A

Jamie struggles with his writing and produces a 40 000 word thesis, but never really feels that he was on top of the task. He leaves the writing to last, and faces problems remembering the key literature that was available at the time he commenced, and so has had to start all over again. Nevertheless he produces some interesting results that are worth reporting. His supervisors provided a lot of feedback on his drafts, much of it expressing concern that the messages were a bit vague. Jamie does his best to address these concerns. The thesis is sent to two reviewers, one internal to the university and the other external to the university. The feedback from the thesis reviewers is however quite negative. Both recommend substantial revision and re-submission, and send in long lists of questions they had. Much of their concerns are about 'woolly' conceptualising of the research questions and one suggests that the data had been over-interpreted. Jamie is very disappointed with the verdict and decides not to bother with the thesis any further, but his supervisors talk him into deferring any such decision for a few weeks at least. The supervisors reassure him that some of the difficulty was due to his research spanning medicine, education and psychology, and the need to reflect the differences of three professions and be clear about how to conduct research at their conjunction. Jamie now wishes that he had paid more attention earlier to learning more about research methods! He accepts this advice (rather reluctantly) and returns to clinical work, initially not even thinking about the research. After a few weeks however, he re-reads the reviewer feedback and the thesis and finds himself understanding many of their concerns. He realises that he could have made his work clearer, and now recognises that he probably should not have commenced a masters degree without some prior research training. In particular, his undergraduate medical research exposure was almost all about biomedical research, and yet his research had combined quantitative and qualitative methods, and he had no real knowledge of qualitative methods.

After a further two months of quiet reflection he decides that he is ready to revise the thesis and get it right. He contacts his supervisors, who are support-ive. He re-reads books on research methodology (including education and psychology research) and revises his description of what he did and why. He also revises his analysis and interpretation and, more importantly, re-writes some sections. The result is a much clearer thesis. This is sent back to both reviewers who applaud the amendments and make relatively brief lists of issues that might be addressed, but suggesting a pass without further formal review.

Case B

Ahmed writes a 20 000 word thesis and a modified version of a commercially available software package that supports decision-making in the patient flow management process, based on clinical algorithms. A CD containing this program is included as an appendix to the thesis. He tailored the program personally, as he has developed quite strong IT skills. The thesis goes to two reviewers, one internal to the university and the other external. Both review-ers suggest amendments to the thesis, one leaving this up to the supervisors to manage, and the other suggesting a need for further review after specific issues had been addressed. The main concern of the second reviewer was that the program on the CD was difficult to follow, even with a strong clinical nursing background. Ahmed and his supervisors meet to discuss this and feel that the problem is more with the instructions that accompanied the software, which they now recognise as being at the level of a person with strong IT skills. They therefore revise the instructions to make them much more user-friendly. The graduate research office sends the revised thesis and CD back to the second reviewer, who now recommends a pass grade.

Case C

Susan writes a 70 000 word thesis and attaches the validated test as an appen-dix. The thesis is sent to three reviewers, one internal to the university, the others external and international. Their feedback is very positive, with one reviewer grading the thesis as 'a clear pass, no amendments needed', and the other two making suggestions for amendments, but recommending that these could be addressed in-house without further formal review. Susan and her supervisors read these suggestions carefully, and feel that some good points had been made, and so revise the thesis to address them. They feel that the result is in fact a stronger thesis. The revised thesis is sent back to the graduate research office and arrangements are made for her graduation at the next graduation ceremony.

Conclusion

It can be a mistake to focus too much and too early on the precise assessment requirements of a research degree. Research training should be approached in the spirit of learning what can be learned from an interesting, potentially exciting, period of candidature, adopting a more self-directed pathway. However, research students and supervisors must know and understand early what the assessment criteria and standards are, so that the research plan can be designed to take students to the correct endpoint of the chosen pathway, however flexible it may be *en route*. Assessment of research training achievement is in principle similar to the assessment of any training programme: there is formative assessment, summative assessment, and in-training assessment. The assessment methods should match the learning objectives and tasks of research training. Research students should invest time in studying the assessment requirements of their particular university and course.

Chapter 8

Communicating research outcomes

If I set out to prove something, I am no real scientist – I have to learn to follow where the real facts lead me – I have to learn to whip my prejudices.

Lazaro Spallanzano 1729–99 (attributed)

Spreading the word

Communicating research outcomes lies at the heart of academic endeavour, because it contributes to improved knowledge and understanding and guides further research. Many research students will be happy that they have achieved the level of communication required for assessment against the requirements of their degree, such as the thesis or other research product. However, the bigger the project and the higher the level of the degree, the more likely it is that research outcomes will be worth communicating beyond the basic requirements to the broader research community. This may be beneficial to both the advancement of research in the particular field of interest and to the academic careers of the research graduates. For graduates with successful projects that are worth reporting, the most important question is not *if* wider reporting is a good idea, but *what, how* and *when* to report research project outcomes more widely than through the degree requirements. There are many ways of achieving this and this chapter discusses the most common methods.

Reporting research outcomes

The question is: what kind of report? Just as there are many kinds of research, each with its own advantages and methods, there are also many ways to report research findings. These range from informal discussions with peers through to formal academic reporting methods. While academics may try to formally publish everything, including things that are not worth the effort, because of a 'publish or perish' culture; inexperienced researchers may feel content to have simply completed their goal and found an answer (or not!), and are less interested in formal processes. Research students often think about reporting results rather late, or perhaps not at all. Instead, they are focused on the here and now of doing their research. One important role of the supervision panel is to ensure that reporting processes are included in the project plan and timelines.

In preparing a report, there are several issues to consider. Is there something to report? If so, why? Who is the most appropriate target audience? How and when should this be reported? Should there be a conference paper, a peer-reviewed journal paper, a monograph or a book? How does the writing fit in with writing a thesis and moving on after the research training is completed? Whose name should be on the product? This chapter attempts to provide simple answers to these questions.

What is there to report?

There should always be something worth reporting from a research project, whether it goes well or badly. The report might be about the answering of the research question, and therefore an expansion of knowledge and understanding. There may also be findings about research methodology, such as what methods appeared to work best in answering the research question. These are of interest to the research community and their reporting is a valuable part of the cycle of discovery, so long as the research design was appropriate, its implementation was as planned, and the analysis and findings were appropriate.

There is a bias in acceptance of reports towards those that have clear positive results – that is, that the research question has been answered, resulting in new knowledge and understanding. Researchers contribute to this bias by not wanting to write about what could be perceived as a research 'failure', and journal editors make assumptions that the research community is more interested in what 'succeeds'. Hence the academic literature has an in-built bias towards reports of clear, expected research findings. This is a pity, because researchers should also be able to discover what does not work, as this can reduce repetition of research ideas that have not been supported and guide improved research design of future projects.

Research that was poorly conceived, based on the wrong literature, or poorly done should not, and probably will not, be reported widely. Such an outcome is a disaster for researchers and research students, but should not happen if the research supervision panel does its job.

Who is the most appropriate target audience?

There can be more than one potential audience for a research report, and this is particularly so for research that is applied to health professional contexts, where there can be several separate, although partially overlapping audiences, depending on the precise nature of the research – the health care practitioners, health care managers, policy makers, regulators and academics. These different groups are likely to require different communication strategies. For example, health care professionals often do not access primary research reports (monographs and academic journals), unless they are in health professional journals, although they may well read abstracts provided in some professional journals. Their interest is in the pithy, digested summary of findings that are relevant to practice, not the detail of how and why. Academics rely on primary research literature that is accessed through international indexing databases (e.g. Medline), and will want to read the detail of the research design, the raw data and the analysis. Managers and regulators will often access a wide variety of communication methods, including the popular media (radio, television and newspapers), and have a preference for large, detailed monographs.

This means that health professionals who are research students may have to produce more than one kind of research report, one each for the key target audiences. In particular, they have a responsibility to produce, in addition to an academic report that meets the criteria for a degree, something that is relevant and accessible to their professional peers, where possible making the outcomes relevant to the professional setting.

What kind of report is most appropriate?

There are several ways of reporting the results of research, as listed in Box 8.1. Deciding which one to aim for requires judgement based on experience, and research supervisors should be best placed to advise. Theses and portfolios were discussed in more detail in Chapter 7, and so are not included in this chapter.

Box 8.1 Kinds of research reports.

Conference poster
Conference oral presentation
Journal paper
Book
Audiovisual media
Electronic media

The first kind of report is a contribution to an appropriate conference of peers, ideally peer reviewed (see below). One form of contribution is a poster presentation, and this can be a very informative process for researchers. Posters are usually grouped by content theme, and if this is done well by the scientific committee then the presentation is to a group of interested and enthusiastic peers. The level of interaction depends on the specific poster presentation format, and is highest when a brief oral presentation is included.

Other forms of conference presentation include oral presentations, seminars, workshops and keynote speeches (generally by invitation), a hierarchy that reflects the degree of difficulty and level of expertise required. Abstract submission processes will provide information on the different categories and what is required. Workshops and seminars usually require a team of contributors, but can be very useful in presenting ideas for further research.

The second form of communicating to an external audience is to publish an article in a refereed journal: this is the traditional academic approach, and careers can be built on a good track record of publishing in certain journals. There are many kinds of journals, and many kinds of journal article. Some journals target narrower professional audiences, and may even be accessible only to that narrow audience in a particular country or region, via professional subscription fees. Others, such as *Science* and *Nature*, aim for a much broader international audience and are available for purchase by anyone. The important question to answer in choosing a journal for submission of an article is: who do I want to read this article? This issue is discussed further below.

The third form of report is a book chapter or a complete book, which is a substantive version of the results and the implications are that it might reach a larger audience that would be prepared to pay for the result. A book chapter requires other authors and editors, but is quite possible when the research result fits in with the work of others around a theme that could be a book. A whole book is much less likely outside humanities research, but is possible when the research project is large and the result of substantial impact and interest. For example, a research project that potentially changes the way in which we view professionalism and leadership in health care may well be substantial and popular enough to justify publication as a book. It is possible that the thesis is very close to a book manuscript, as both are lengthy documents. Books are not necessarily much longer than theses, but require expansion of results, interpretation and relevance to the real world, and contraction or even omission of methodology and detailed results. They also need a publisher, and publishers will not publish a book at their cost unless they can sell enough copies. Most academic books are not big sellers, and therefore carry a high price. Occasionally the research project funder will sponsor a book or equivalent product, particularly if there is potential for a policy or commercial gain.

While books are still in bound paper format rather than electronic (this may well change as ebooks grow in acceptance), equivalent academic products do not need to be the traditional bound paper format, but can be in the form of a CD-ROM, a DVD, a television series, a film or a website. The choice depends on the material and the audience. Supervisors may be best placed to advise on the most appropriate format.

The importance of peer review

Peer review is an important academic concept that is not well understood by novice researchers. While a research project may be based on currently available evidence and literature, the best source of current opinion and judgement is generally to be found in the research community. Currently active researchers are generally ahead of the literature because of their research or intelligence gained through either personal research networks or reviewing of the results of other researchers (paper submissions, grant proposals etc.). Just as it is important to access current researchers in the relevant field when developing a research project, it is important to check with current researchers when interpreting results. Their feedback is generally helpful and it is better to obtain it before completion and submission of any report product so that it will be of the best quality. Theses are marked by peer review (the individuals cannot be those who provided assistance), as are any conference paper, journal article and book submissions, and unexpected comments will be less likely if there has been peer review at an early stage.

While peer review is generally a positive and helpful process, it is possible for it to result in negative, even malicious comments. The reasons for this predominantly relate to poor behaviour by reviewers, from poor matching of expertise through to conflict of interest. Publishers try hard to minimise these situations. Any author who receives negative feedback should share the feedback with other researchers to find out if something really is wrong or missing. If it is, fix it. If the negative or nasty reviewer comments represent a minority view or conflict of interest, the publisher may be interested in receiving that advice.

Indexing journal papers

In academic communication one important issue is the accessibility of the material outside the immediate readership of the chosen journal. This is achieved via electronic databases which list the contents of journals by author, title, subject, key words and themes etc., generally within a few weeks of publication. All these headings are searchable items in a database that is usually web-accessible and therefore available, at least in the form of abstracts, to a much wider audience. Access to full text versions may require journal subscription either directly to the publisher or via a university or professional group subscription. There are several with direct relevance to health care, including MEDLINE, CINAHL (Content Index for Nursing and Allied Health Professions), ERIC (Educational Resources Index Citation) and PSYCHLIT (psychology literature). None of these indexing services include all relevant journals, but instead choose journals on merit, based on the perceived quality of each journal, as measured by the rates of citation of papers in those journals. There is intense competition amongst journals to be listed in a recognised database, the most prestigious of which is MEDLINE, and many journals do not succeed.

Hence any search of only the recognised indexing databases will not identify the whole literature that may be relevant. Increasingly, people use more widely accessible search engines, such as Ingenta, Biomedcentral and Google Scholar, but these may include material that some academics would not regard highly. In particular, it is wise to avoid using the most open search engines, such as Google, for academic purposes, as the results will be less specific and will have no quality filter at all. The other strategy to obtain non-indexed material is to search Government departmental websites for formal reports, which may summarise the literature well and be influential in a policy sense, but will not appear in many indexing databases.

Journal impact factors

Just as being in a recognised citation database indicates a perception of the quality of individual journals, so too does the level of the citation index. The citation index of individual journals reflects the frequency of citation from within indexed databases, and is used to derive an impact factor, expressed as a number from 0 upwards, with the highest around 15. Translating this into meaningful words is difficult, but in summary the higher the impact factor, the more widely recognised the journal.

There is a complex *chicken and egg* problem here, because high recognition leads to a higher impact factor which leads to higher recognition. Many good journals struggle early to achieve a place in the citation index, and so good research published in newer journals may not achieve either a place in an indexing system or recognition by the author's employing university. This means that there is a bias towards certain well established and widely accessible journals that report breakthrough level advances of widespread interest and significance. The relevance of this to researchers is that much of the institutional recognition for academic success comes from publishing a research paper in a refereed academic journal with a high impact factor. This can be difficult to achieve for any researcher, let alone research students. Health professional research students who are researching issues of relevance to their specific professional context have an additional hurdle, because their research results can be so applied to the particular profession that any reporting needs to be back to that broader professional group, via a profession-specific journal that will have a narrow and small audience, and therefore either a low or no impact factor. Journal impact factors are one of the most controversial topics in research, as they are often misunderstood or mis-applied.

Self-publishing

An emerging issue with academic output is who pays for the publication? For journals and books, the traditional view is that a publisher accepts manuscripts, arranges peer review, correction and editing, pays the costs of publishing, then recoups the cost through selling copies and journal subscriptions. However, academic publishing is expensive, as numbers of readers are very small in comparison with mass media markets, and affordability can decrease the capacity to publish all research that may merit dissemination. A recent response to this dilemma is for authors to pay for the journal publication themselves, and make them available free to readers, usually via a web-based journal platform called 'open access' journals. Some universities will pay for the publications, but in most cases the individual authors have to make a contribution. If this trend continues, then perhaps the financial outlay will be the same, as universities currently pay very high journal subscription fees, but accessibility will increase. Self-publication of academic books (the author pays) is increasingly available: some printing companies will also print and bind self-published books, which the author can then sell direct to an audience. However all forms of self-publishing raise concerns about the potential for weak or no peer review to result in lower academic standards. One very controversial issue here is the extent to which publishers might accept payment to publish research that is not worthy of being published. Research supervisors may offer the best advice on which journals and publishers to consider.

Tips on academic writing

Among researchers and research students the level of interest and skill in writing is variable. Many novice researchers will find writing daunting. Some will take a rather utilitarian view, preferring to write simple, concise summaries in a way that matches discipline needs. For example, in bioscience conference papers generally follow the IMRAD format and are heavy on methodology, data and conclusions that contribute to the evidence base. Others might see writing as a creative task that allows messages to be placed within reach of different but relevant audiences, with the aim of provoking debate.

The skills of academic writing improve with experience. The most important tip is to have a message that is worth disseminating, as that will gain an audience. Different professions and disciplines have their own journals, websites and conferences, and authors need to know about these. Different professions and disciplines have different versions of academic style. For example, in bioscience the writing style is more direct, factual, concise and categorised. In the humanities, or where qualitative methods have been used, there is room for discussion and exploration, often resulting in much longer and apparently discursive report products. It is important to follow the relevant publisher's guidelines about word length, formatting, referencing and authorship, or submissions risk being rejected at first base. Referencing can be complex, as there are several different formats and the choice of system may depend on the particular profession or research field. In health research the two common systems are the Vancouver and Harvard systems, but social science literature can use other systems. Journal editors provide author guidelines that make it clear which one to use for papers, and each university will have its own style manual that must be observed. Software packages are available that can take basic referencing information and re-format that information into any of the more common systems. Ask colleagues to read the draft and give feedback, as sometimes authors are so absorbed in their projects that they cannot see gaps in logic or flow. It is wise to seek feedback from someone who does not know anything about the research or even the topic, as such a person can provide more general advice about 'readability' and interest. Finally, do not give up easily if a publisher or journal editor says no. Although rejections are disappointing, read the feedback carefully, as it is often accurate. Try to correct fixable flaws and submit elsewhere. These tips are summarised in Box 8.2.

Box 8.2 Tips on academic writing.

- Have something to say that is worth reading or hearing
- Be familiar with your professional reporting outlets
- Identify the most likely audience
- Work out the most relevant conference/journal/publisher
- Understand and follow conference/journal/publishers' guidelines
- Understand and follow discipline-based academic style conventions
- Select and observe consistently the appropriate referencing system
- Start by just putting into words whatever comes to mind
- Have colleagues read drafts and give feedback
- Ensure careful editing and proof reading
- Be prepared to be persistent

Writing for more than one product

While some find writing fun, the most efficient way of approaching the writing of more than one form of research report (e.g. a thesis, a conference presentation and a journal paper) is to write them at the same time. This does not mean literally the writing of three separate pieces concurrently, but rather planning the writing of more than one report product as a longer version that can be trimmed and edited to be another report product. This requires planning, but is not difficult, as a thesis requires a lot of information that need not be in shorter report products. Hence some thesis sections are simply omitted, while others are summarised versions of the longer product text. A further complication is that different products can require different formatting, styles and referencing systems. The referencing software mentioned above can be very helpful. This kind of writing for multiple products can be difficult for novice researchers, but the skill can develop with experience.

Authorship rules

Authorship is a potentially complex and controversial issue, although in principle it is simple. Not long ago every research report from university departments would include the name of the head of that department as an author, even if he or she personally had nothing to do with the research project. This would now be regarded as academic misconduct, taking more credit than was due through exploitation of more junior staff and research students. The current view is that all contributors to academic output should be recognised in a manner that reflects their role.

With current trends towards multi-professional and multi-institution research collaboration, there may be a large number of contributors, so exactly how individual contributors are acknowledged can appear complex. This issue should be discussed with supervisors early in the project. If there are any local institutional guidelines, find them and use them as a starting point in the discussion. If there are no local guidelines, consider the more general rules of academic authorship that are summarised in Box 8.3. These may however be modified, depending on the precise field of research.

Box 8.3 General rules of authorship.

1 Authorship rights are earned by individuals making a significant contribution to the project. Ideally this contribution is during several or all stages of the project.

2 The order of authorship should reflect the relative contribution of individuals to the project. Those with the greatest contribution are usually listed early.

3 First authorship should go to the individual who made a major contribution, ideally including at least a contribution to writing the report or paper.

4 Individuals who made smaller contributions may be acknowledged formally either before or after the substantive text.

5 Current practice is moving towards listing all contributors with a description of their precise contribution.

One important issue is the order of authorship, as this may suggest relative importance of contributions, although there are subtle differences in this interpretation, depending on the field of research. Generally speaking, novice researchers may start off as a last author, with their supervisors first, and then move up the list to be first authors when they lead research projects. However in some research fields novice researchers often go first, particularly when they have done most of the work, and supervisors go last. In measuring academic cv of individuals in those research fields, appointment panels may interpret the observation that experienced researchers are often last author as evidence of desirable research supervision experience. It is best to seek advice on this from supervisors and fellow research students.

There are some differences here between the situations of recent undergraduate students and more experienced professionals. The former is more likely to join a team with ready-made projects, and so is less likely to play a significant part in all stages of a project. The original concept, the literature review, the research question and the methods will probably already be largely worked out, leaving the research student as the apprentice who will play a stronger role in data collection and interpretation, learning from assisting their supervisors. Such contributions result in less recognition in communicating outcomes, although ideally supervisors will 'give' responsibility for part of the project, particularly at PhD level, and that can allow for higher recognition rights for that part of the project.

For experienced health professionals, the original concept and general research question is more likely to have come from them. Supervisors will play very important roles in refining the question, advising on literature and selecting methods, but the student is then more likely to personally perform much of the work. The professional context may be crucial to the research, and the student may be the primary source. Hence for more experienced professionals who become research students, much more of the intellectual property is theirs, and this should be recognised. It is more common for these students to be first authors in conference presentations and papers.

Emerging current practice in many reporting outlets is to describe the precise roles of each of the listed contributors. For some journals this is not provided in the text, due to space limitations, but may be part of the submission process that all authors must sign. Although this may seem to be a long-winded approach, it has the clear advantage of making contributions absolutely explicit. An example is provided in Box 8.4.

Box 8.4 An example of current authorship practice.

ABC conducted the initial literature, framed the research question, contributed to development of the methods and wrote the first draft of this paper. DEF led the development of the research methods and reviewed drafts of the paper. GHI provided research supervision and contributed to data analysis and reviewing drafts. JKL assisted in recruitment of subjects and reviewing drafts of the paper.

Case studies

Our three research students have been busy for several months or years, and are nearing completion of their research training projects.

Case A

Jamie recovers his self esteem and feels satisfaction that he has achieved what he set out to achieve, even if by a rockier and longer route than intended. He is happy with the professional recognition he has gained for his work, and accepts an invitation to sit on an advisory committee that is considering how to detect and manage poorly performing doctors. He also writes from his thesis the paper that was suggested by an academic at a conference, and after some revision in response to reviewers' comments, it has been accepted. He finds the journal review process to be similar but easier than that of his thesis, although the task of writing in 1500 words a summary of the 40 000 words was more difficult than he expected.

Case B

Ahmed is keen to develop further his software management system. His employer has been very supportive in the development and trialling of the software, and has offered to implement the program and further trial it. The management academic points out that if all goes well there is the potential for some form of a commercial result by which Ahmed and his supervisors might earn a small amount of money from their intellectual property. Ahmed presents the software at an emergency medicine conference and is asked to write a paper for an emergency medicine journal. It is agreed that he will be the first author, the management academic the second author and the replacement nurse academic supervisor the third author. The original nurse academic supervisor has had very little to do with the project and is happy to stand out of this development.

Case C

Susan's project is very successful, resulting in a validated and benchmarked test for her intended target audience. Susan writes two journal papers based on her thesis, one each for a professional and an educational measurement journal. She is invited to write a chapter for a new book on the educational assessment of adolescents, being edited by the internationally noted researchers who gave her advice early in the project and stayed in contact throughout. After a well-received conference paper many of her colleagues are keen to adopt her version of the test, and the test publisher is negotiating to incorporate her modifications, most likely on a commercial basis.

Conclusion

Appropriate reporting of the results of research projects is an essential part of each project, and is an important part of academic life. This activity should not be driven by a 'publish or perish' mentality, bur rather a conceptual framework of contributing to the knowledge and evidence base within the relevant academic and professional literature. Research report products generally require academic writing skills, although the format must conform to the various professional and discipline-based conventions and may increasingly be electronic rather than paper-based. Recognition of contributors should be discussed and agreed early. Research students should take advice from their supervisors about possible publishing options, and should consider multiple reporting products, as relevant to the profession and format. Academic writing skills will improve with experience.

Chapter 9

What next?

A clinician is complex. He is part practical scientist, and part historian.

Thomas Addis 1881–1949

The end or the beginning?

The completion of a research project can mean many things. One outcome is a feeling of relief, as it will be the end of a busy period that brought complexity and hard work. Other priorities in life can now resume prominence, whether they are work or family activities or, most likely, a combination of the two. Another outcome is a sense of reward for the effort, as successful research students receive degrees and public recognition. Degree ceremonies can be really happy events, with family, friends and colleagues able to share in the success and receive their due recognition. Reading your own name in a publication for the first time can be quite a thrill, as it proves that someone else really is interested in the results of the research.

Strangely enough, a third outcome can be a sense of emptiness and uncertainty. What should I do next? Should I go back to being a full-time clinician? Should I have a long break from work? Should I focus on family priorities? Should I do some more research, perhaps following up my recent project? None of these options is right or wrong, and the decision has to be made by the individual, ideally in consultation with family and friends. Whatever choice is made, the period of research training candidature should contribute to a more interesting next phase in life.

Applied professional practice

One very attractive option for health professionals with a research degree is a return to professional practice, where the results of the research can ideally be applied. Where the research is directly related to clinical or education practice, the individual is likely to develop into, and be recognised as, a leader in the area of expertise. Even where the research is not directly relevant to any specific field of professional practice, completion of a research degree should mean that graduates possess an improved range of generic skills that may be very useful in professional practice, including: framing more precise questions that are relevant to practice; information gathering strategies; information analysis; synthesis of ideas and concepts; and communication strategies. It is generally, although not necessarily, true that the higher the level of research training, the higher is the acquisition of these skills.

All of these skills are useful in any work context, particularly where important decisions are to be made, as is the norm in health professional practice. Patient care poses questions about the best way to proceed, and academic training should improve the ability to frame more precise questions to guide the process of answering them. The academic approach to gathering relevant information is broad, seeking a range of sources, from the more accessible to the least accessible, and includes going directly to identifiable experts. The analysis of that information can use the methods learned in research, both quantitative and qualitative, depending on the nature of the information. Qualitative thematic analysis skills can be particularly helpful in dealing with complex debates. Bringing ideas and concepts together is part of writing both the literature review and the discussion sections in the research report. Finally, communication strategies are learned through conference presentations, writing research reports and use of audio-visual media. These skills can contribute to an improvement in health care and patient outcomes, and may lead the practitioner into professional leadership roles.

Academic careers

Many research students will at some stage look back and feel that the period of research was one of the more exciting and dynamic phases of their lives. The sooner this happens, the more likely is a desire to continue research activity at some time. There are two ways of achieving this goal. The first is as a predominantly professional practitioner, maintaining a part-time involvement in academic life through continuing research, usually in collaboration with academic colleagues. This can be a very satisfying career pathway, providing greater freedom and autonomy, as it allows for greater individual choice of when to pursue what part of a career. As research opportunities wax and wane, or as interest dictates, the proportion of time devoted to clinical practice and to research can vary. It is however very difficult to devote enough time to the research part of the career to establish a more permanent senior research career.

The second pathway is that of the career academic researcher, an individual who will work for a university (or similar research institution) and attempt to pursue research ideas or a research agenda to an advanced stage of discovery and/or understanding. These are the people who are more likely to follow the traditional junior researcher–senior researcher–research supervisor–research dean– vice-chancellor pathway, although very few want to enter serious full-time management roles. One of the more significant problems faced by career researchers is what to do after a successful career. It is very hard to stay at the edge of discovery for very long, and huge breakthroughs are rare. Research lifestyles can be difficult to fit in with other commitments, as there will be periods of frenetic, often creative activity, periods pre-occupied with more mundane activity, all driven by a combination of opportunity, networks and sometimes luck. More experienced researchers share some of the work-life balance challenges faced by their research students, and even seniority does not guarantee a predictable work life in research.

Research performance is now so linked to measures such as external grants, publications and invited lectures that there is less room towards the top for respected, senior colleagues who no longer bring in income and prestige. While research careers can be an amazing ride, the choice of exits can be restricted for those who do not stay on the A list. Some will develop an interest in management, which in universities is now a complex and highly professional role that requires preparation and training, while others might increase their teaching commitment, although good researchers are by no means necessarily good teachers. Happily, for academic health professionals, most combine academic and clinical practice throughout their careers and can vary the proportion of clinical, teaching and research activity as careers evolve.

Commercialising intellectual property

Most research is conducted in the more established tradition of working from and contributing back to a body of shared knowledge that is 'owned' in the public interest by humanity. This is all a bit vague, but this usually does not matter because few research discoveries are easily converted to commercial products that will earn income for either individual researchers or their employing universities. There are of course important examples where there is a commercial product, and universities are becoming better at exploiting such opportunities, often through partnerships with established companies or the development of their own 'spin off' commercial ventures. Pharmaceutical companies are an example of a whole sector of industry that feeds off and contributes to research that is turned into often expensive drugs, many of which make significant contributions to an improvement in the quality of health care. Competition is intense and secrecy is the norm until discoveries are patented. On the other hand, there is a recent example of collaboration of several research groups to map the human genome which, although a huge scientific outcome with substantial commercial potential, was considered to be best shared to facilitate faster and further applied research that in itself might be commercially important.

It is unlikely, but not impossible, that a student research project will produce a commercially successful product. It is more likely that a student project might make a contribution to a chain of research activities that might end up with a product that might have commercial potential. Rights will be guided by the early discussions on intellectual property and authorships rules, as well as rules of the particular university. Where any commercial value appears to be possible, students and their supervisors should discuss the issue early and seek formal advice from their university.

Case studies

Our three research students have all graduated, and are considering what to do next.

Case A

Jamie can now look back on his research training as an ultimately positive experience. He now feels much more confident and competent in his role as an educator. He is interested in doing some follow up research, but cannot face the thought of re-immersion in research too soon. In particular, he wants to wait until his children are older and for his partner, also a busy career person, to have an opportunity to pursue some mid-career professional development. He is offered, and accepts, a more leading role in the educational programme, and arranges his work so that he can manage both that and still a substantial share of the clinical workload. This is easier because his partners have got used to his absence for research, and the practice roster was working well with the addition of a part-time GP. Jamie finds a combination of clinical and educational practice to be very interesting and rewarding, but recognises the challenge of balancing those two interests, and he does not think that any more formal academic career development is needed at this stage.

Case B

Ahmed has his masters degree, and has developed greater confidence in both his clinical practice and his ability to manage the triaging of sporting injuries. Although thrilled that his employer is so supportive and will trial the results of his project, he is developing a thirst to take this further. His supervisors recommend that he use the extension to other hospitals to enrol in a PhD that would evaluate the further development. Ahmed is considering this, although feels he should return to clinical nursing full-time for a while first.

Case C

Susan appears to have attained both national and international recognition for her research, as there is wider interest in using the test she has validated and benchmarked. She seeks legal and commercial advice on how to deal with the approach to commercialise the test. As the idea was mostly hers, she finds that she is in a position to sign agreements that might earn her some income, depending on the success of the commercialisation. She is also invited to apply for posts as a lecturer at three universities, one in North America. Her partner and children are thrilled at her success, but do not want to move to North America! She is considering how to manage a more academic career, still including professional practice, and with the likelihood of additional income from sales of her test.

Conclusion

Research training can provide graduates with a set of useful and transferable generic skills that should be useful in professional practice, and can open up interesting career possibilities. Most health professionals who attain research degrees will continue to combine professional practice with some academic role, and may well have increased flexibility to shape their career. Ultimately, research training degrees are just one way of enhancing professional life, but should be considered by those with an interest in answering questions that arise from professional practice.

Index